Complete
Dental Assistant's,
Secretary's, and Hygienist's
Handbook

Complete
Dental Assistant's,
Secretary's, and Hygienist's
Handbook

Charles A. Reap, Jr., D.D.S.

Parker Publishing Company, Inc.

West Nyack, New York

Library of Congress Cataloging in Publication Data

Reap, Charles A
   Complete dental assistant's, secretary's, and
hygienist's handbook.

   1. Dental assistants--Handbooks, manuals, etc.
2. Dental hygienists--Handbooks, manuals, etc.
I. Title. [DNLM: 1. Dental assistants. 2. Dental
hygienists. WU 90 R288c 1973]
RK60.5.R4   651'.9'6176   72-12789
ISBN 0-13-159855-4

Printed in the United States of America

This book is dedicated to

my wife Betty
and my children Ellen, Cindy,
Linda, Chuck and Hunter,

whose patience and understanding are
deeply appreciated.

A Word from the Author About This Book

One of the keys to the successful practice of dentistry is that old but appropriate word—"teamwork." In days past this was not really so very important, as the dentist most frequently was capable of working alone, or at least with a bare minimum of assistance. He simply used his lone assistant to clean up his instruments after he had completed his work for his patient, or to answer the telephone and perhaps to prepare and mail the monthly statements. If he was really advanced for his time, he might let his assistant hand him an instrument occasionally. But as the other saying goes, "them days is gone forever!"

In today's modern, fast-moving world it is practically impossible for any dentist to practice truly successful dentistry without a capable assistant. In reality she has evolved into more of an "associate," than an "assistant." If the dentist can only know when and how to use his dental auxiliary as effectively as possible, he can easily expand his scope to an almost unlimited amount.

The purpose of this writing is twofold. First, primarily to help you, the dental auxiliary, to become better qualified and better trained, so that you will become a stronger member of the dental team. Second, it will help you to help the dentist learn to use your skills and knowledge to a far better degree than ever before.

This book is not a primer. It is directed to the dental assistant who already has learned and developed some basic skills in the field. It is not aimed at teaching the basics of dentistry, but rather should be considered a postgraduate course for the dental auxiliary.

7

If you are relatively new to our profession, I suggest you read and reread each chapter until you practically know it by heart, and then apply its principles to your own doctor's practice. Naturally your dentist will practice his type of dentistry somewhat differently from another man, so adaptation is a key word.

If you consider yourself an old-timer with us, then I recommend that you read each chapter and section diligently and with an open mind as to how you can use various hints and tips that I have given you. Use the margins liberally for notes and your own ideas. Underline important sections for easy recall later. Then every few months, thumb casually through the book to perhaps catch again that spark that will open up new vistas of knowledge and excitement for you.

One theme that you will find continually coming through to you in this book is the point that you, as a dental auxiliary, should help your dentist to utilize your services and abilities. By this I mean that many dentists simply do not know quite how to use you as an assistant. They may see a particular problem, but may not have the answer. You should be able to anticipate such difficulties and suggest to your doctor that you might do this, or do that, in order to be of more assistance.

Communications breakdown is frequently a problem in the daily workings of the busy dental office. A dentist may note a particular problem now, but be so busy as to delay its discussion until later, and then forget to mention it when he has the time. Then the end result of all of this is that the dentist just goes along and continues with things not really quite like he would prefer them to be. Thus, teamwork either from his side or the side of the dental assistant suffers. Therefore, it behooves the competent dental assistant to guard against this result as much as possible, or at least try to head things off. So, as you read this book, think of your own practice and of the many, many things you can see that might potentially be a problem.

You will find the "office conference" mentioned in this book several times. These have proven to be worth their weight in gold in practices throughout the country. It is here that potential "bugs" can be headed off in advance and better methods of teamwork can be perfected. It is also here that the real "guts" of a practice can be analyzed and better goals can be sighted and aimed for.

So, finally, my suggestions to you would be these: read the book and think out ways that you can apply its suggestions to your own individual practice. Suggest to your dentist that *he* read it also, and then both of you sit down and thoroughly discuss any ideas you have come to that you feel may benefit all concerned. This way you will also develop skills in thinking out solutions to specific problems as they arise in your office, and with the teamwork concepts that follow, you all will surely build and help build some of the country's outstanding dental practices.

As this book is being written the entire profession seems to be on the very threshold of new and exciting realms of change. Expanded duties for the dental auxiliary seem to be the key and can be looked forward to with eager eyes by all who care for the very best in dentistry. One thing that is not yet clear is just how far dentistry can go in permitting dental auxiliaries to take over traditional tasks. The profession must consider its obligation to its patients first and foremost. The correction of dental disease by the best possible means is necessary, but many in the profession tend to feel that anyone with less than a D.D.S. or D.M.D. should not be allowed to perform dental procedures on patients. On the other hand, there seems to be no other way out for the dental profession if it is going to treat all of the patients who need and desire its help.

Until the problem is resolved, it will behoove the dental assistant, secretary, and hygienist to constantly maintain and try to improve their knowledge and capabilities in dentistry.

Charles A. Reap, Jr., D.D.S.

Contents

part 1

The Secretarial

Assistant

1 | Key Points for Success in Your Office

The Importance of Accuracy

Webster defines the term "accuracy" as "the quality or state of being careful and exact, free from errors, precise." It is just in this manner that your dentist-employer relies on you. You must be free from error at all times. There is simply no room for anyone in a dental office who continually makes mistakes. The old saying, "To err is human, to forgive divine," simply does not apply here.

Whenever you are working with a person's health as we are in dentistry, errors can become disastrous. A simple error in the direction of a high-speed bur of as much as one-quarter of a millimeter can mean the life or death of a tooth. The loss of a tooth can alter the entire personality of a person for a lifetime.

Take a look into the business and financial world. Imagine what complications and confusion can occur if a single decimal point is misplaced by a banking institution. One might wonder how you might feel if, next payday, your check reads $10,000.

Certainly reams and reams have been written about the problems that have developed when a bank made an error and added an account wrong, compounding the original error by thousands.

So it is in dentistry. We are in the business world, and as such, we must continually search out any possible errors and eliminate them. All of our addition and substraction must be accurate. It is so simple to add six and seven and arrive at thirteen. It can be so much trouble to add it on the adding machine, when you know it by heart anyway. But you must remember this: there is always the one time when you were adding these figures, and suddenly the phone rang, or a patient walked in, and you had already been adding similar figures for several minutes, and now, this time, you record fourteen. It can be so simple an error as to go practically unnoticed, but there it is. And no other calculations that have any relationship with this figure will be accurate. If this were to be the daily production or collection figures for your doctor at the early part of the month, then this error might well go unnoticed until the end-of-the-month audit. Then the accountant would have to go back over some thirty calculations in order to correct an error of only one!

Practically all the fees we work with in the profession are in whole dollars. At least this eliminates two figures as sources of errors. But pity on the dental assistant when the telephone rings on that hectic Monday morning after sending out statements, and the doctor just happens to answer the phone, and Mrs. Special Patient had found that *you* inadvertently added her bill wrong and charged her one dollar too much!

Does your doctor deduct the amount in error from your pay check if you added up his estimates wrong on Mr. Brown's case, and the estimate was fifty dollars short of the normal fee? What would you do if you were in his shoes?

How does it make your employer feel if you accidentally made an error and appointed two different patients for the same time? And the doctor just happens to walk into the business office when both patients are showing you that they both have cards? And they both insist on being seen? And they both need to be seen? A simple error of omitting one patient's name from the appointment book certainly became compounded quickly, didn't it?

How would it make you feel—inside—if you accidentally

mixed a ZOE paste when the doctor had asked for a calcium hydroxide paste for a pulpal exposure; he did not know the difference, because they both look the same, and the patient lost the tooth–due to your carelessness? The patient would not know it was your fault, nor would the doctor, but could you live with it?

Could you live well if you made the error of giving your doctor a syringe loaded with an anesthetic containing a drug that the patient had expressed allergic reactions to and the doctor didn't catch it, and the patient died? Think about it. Just a small error. Small.

Let's face it, there is really no such thing as a small error, is there? Each and every incorrect thing you do creates troubles. Even if you find the mistake immediately, and correct it, it took a moment of your time, didn't it? And every second counts in the average dental office. Efficiency is the maxim, and efficiency means minimized wasted time, which in turn means *no errors.*

In summary, please Miss Dental Assistant, try to become that perfect someone who never makes mistakes. Always concentrate on making every move count, and in making every move the correct one. If you find yourself repeating mistakes, the same ones over and over, then immediately pinpoint the cause of the problem and eliminate it. Let correctness become your motto.

How to Keep Your Enthusiasm

In any job or profession or even any phase of everyday living, enthusiasm and your zest for living can occasionally wear thin and wane. It follows that if one has no happiness in the job she is doing, then that job can become a horrible chore. It can affect your relationship with your employer, your patients, your friends, and can even alter your personality.

Nothing can create more disillusionment to a prospective new patient than to call a dental office, and hear the dental secretary on the line, with a dull, bored, cheerless voice, that says in effect, "I'm bored to death with it all, and I wish I were somewhere else, and you hadn't bothered to call." Well, if you have this attitude, don't worry, pretty soon you will be elsewhere, and you will not be bored with this job–you will not have it!

You, as the dental secretary, are the first contact the average patient has with the dental office. It is here that first impressions of the office are made, and it is you who must create the image of a fine, wholesome personality. This exuberance must always be present. It is part of your job, and if it is not there, you are not following through with the tasks for which you were hired.

I realize that doing the same job day after day, month after month, and year after year, cannot help but become somewhat routine after a while. After all, you see about the same faces every day, and frequently hear practically the same things all day long. How can you remain cheerful at all times?

The secret is enthusiasm! I have never met a person who was enthusiastic about a particular subject who was not exciting to talk to. This enthusiasm is contagious, and can quickly spread to others. This is what can stir one's blood. It therefore becomes vital that every patient who speaks to you—every time—becomes well aware of your zest for life, your inner happiness, your enthusiasm. Just talking to you will make every patient feel better, and be happier. This will in turn create more confidence in your office.

But how does one keep his enthusiasm month after month when the job is so repetitious?

The best solution is to continually create projects. If you were constantly working toward a goal, then you would continually be in the throes of excitement and expectation. This helps to arouse the enthusiasm we all need.

Each month have a goal to work toward, and also one each year. You may even wish to have a daily goal. Then, as you see yourself arriving at that goal, set a higher one next time. If your goal is a certain financial figure, make sure it is set high enough to create a drive. If it is set too low, and too easily reached, there will be a certain lack of drive. On the other hand, make sure it is not set so high as to seem impossible and unreachable, since this will likely have the oposite effect, and create disillusionment, and the resultant sour personality.

Your projects can be many other things besides financial. Here you can let your imagination run wild. Look around your office. Do you see any potential projects to work on or any unfinished tasks that were started months ago, and just sort of dropped?

Go out into the reception room when no patients are there. Sit down in each seat, and look around the room with the eye of the new patient. Do you see any areas that do not look neat? Can you rearrange the furniture in any fashion that will enhance the comfort or convenience of the office or patients? How about switching the pictures from one wall to another? Perhaps you can talk the doctor into buying new lampshades for the lamps. This can practically give you a new reception room simply by altering two lampshades with new colors and shapes. See how easy it is to find new projects! If you have only one new project a month, it will help to create hours of enthusiasm.

Follow this same procedure throughout the entire office and look into each nook and cranny for ways to alter the physical surroundings. Do not look for ways to spend the doctor's money—he has expenses enough as it is. But if you do decide on something that will definitely create a valuable asset to the office, you can at least find out exactly what you want, and where it can be purchased, and how much it will cost. Then present this in a formal fashion to your dentist and let him decide for himself whether or not he wishes to proceed with it. He may not decide to follow through, but you can bet he will respect your ideas and persistence in having all of the information available to him.

Why not look inward? How about a few self-improvement projects for yourself? How long has it been since you changed your hair-do? If you have a particular reason for not altering it, it may well pay you to look into the various types—and colors—of wigs and hairpieces now available at reasonable prices. You could give your employer a "new" secretary every week. Certainly the same old uniforms day after day can become monotonous for all those people around you. Perhaps it will be just fine with your doctor if you change to colors. There are many neat and professional pastel uniforms on the market today. A recent survey asked dental patients what they thought of colored uniforms on the dental assistants as compared to the standard white ones. The original concern was that they might feel the uniforms pointed too much to the occupation of waitress or hairdresser. The most common response on the survey—"friendly!" No doubt, the white stockings, the cap, the professional attitude set the dental auxiliary apart from the other occupations.

For more continuing projects, let your imagination be your

only limitation. You and the other auxiliaries in the office, and even the doctor can take a lunch hour occasionally and have a "brainstorming" session. This is when you all just "let yourselves go" in imagination. Have someone record all ideas mentioned, freely mentioning anything that may come into your heads that might possibly—no matter how remotely—improve the office staff, facilities, and operations. You might well get fifty to one hundred ideas in just a half-hour or so. Now many of these ideas may not turn into anything useful, but on the other hand, many will, and then you have projects for a while.

My basic point is this: keep thinking—all the time—for various gimmicks, thoughts, projects—anything that you will want to follow through on that will help to create and keep enthusiasm in your dental office. Things will just naturally go better this way.

Shortcuts to the Happier Day

A person is happiest when he can look back and see accomplishment. If you can know in your own mind that today you have been a real asset to something or someone, then you automatically will have a special degree of happiness. It then follows that you must continually create ways to accomplish things.

The worst thing in your day is likely to be the onset of boredom from repetition. Much of your life is repetition, but it is unlikely you are bored with it. Another frequent problem is the unpleasant chore—the chore you dread, either because it is unpleasant to you, or else simply because it offers you absolutely no challenge. Someone once said, "the shortest answer is doing the thing." This means to go ahead and jump headlong into that which you find most distasteful and get it over with. In this manner at least you will not find yourself sitting around dreading it and remaining unhappy the entire time. Always do that thing first that you'd rather not do at all, and you will be a happier person.

It has often been said, "Happiness is derived from helping others." Where else can you find a better occupation or profession than dentistry? Every single thing we do in our business has something or another to do with helping others. The basic fact that we actually *create* good health, and continually preach prevention is certainly reasonable enough knowledge from which to derive inner pleasure.

But certainly, one must derive pleasure from helping others in the many other ways possible. Why not create for yourself a permanent smile? This smile then will be available for all to see. Can you honestly look at someone who gives you a sincere, pleasant smile, and not feel better? The smile itself is such a simple thing, yet it can immediately put even the most fearsome, grouchy patient at ease. And isn't it nice to have only pleasant patients in your reception room? Just a simple smile works wonders. A famous writer once declared, "The smile that lights the face will also warm the heart." Please do not ever forget to be pleasant.

How to Create the World's Nicest Patients

One of your goals as a postgraduate professional must surely be to create and maintain the most agreeable patients possible— nice people who will actually look forward to coming into the office and seeing you, and in turn the doctor. You are, after all, the first face they are likely to see when they enter. In order to insure their one hundred percent loyalty to your office, and their best understanding when things might go awry, it is most helpful to have these people happy with the practice.

The basic thought? Consideration of the feelings of others. If you will develop the simple gesture of offering some kindness to each and every patient who enters your reception room, it will not be long before the results begin to pay off. This may possibly sound somewhat crass and commercial, but the true spirit of being thoughtful is always in good style wherever you may go. As I have repeatedly tried to emphasize, though, you must be sincere. Never let any patient even begin to think that you are simply being nice because the boss said to be nice, or that it is simply part of your job.

You can begin your new approach by learning and remembering the patients' names. We all like to feel that we are important enough in someone else's mind to have them remember us. How about this? "Why, hello, Mary Helen. How are you today?" Isn't this much better than even a cheery "Good morning!" These same old "Good morning" and "Good afternoon" greetings can be heard in every business and professional establishment worth its salt in the country. Why don't you be the one bright spot in their day, and say something a little different—something with an individual flavor to it—something to let this patient know you are really interested in him as a person, not just another patient in the daily long line of patients.

You certainly will have some difficulty getting to know a new patient, his likes and dislikes, but you will, or course, greet each patient with a warm hello. Tell him who you are and that we are glad to see (meet) him, and that the doctor will see him in just a few moments.

Can you take his coat and hang it up for him? Offer him coffee? Make sure he will have enough time to drink at least half a cup before the doctor is ready to see him. It is not a very nice feeling to have coffee offered, then taken away after your first sip.

Does your doctor have a refrigerator available in the office? Why not offer iced tea in the summer? The patients love it. If you have no refrigerator available, you can always pick up a bag of crushed ice at a local store, and store it in a styrofoam chest in the lab. It is only a little trouble, but can create some very pleasant thoughts on the part of your patients.

After you have known your patients a while, you should be able to pick up little items about their likes and dislikes, their pleasures, their hobbies, their pets, their traveling experiences, and many similar things. You will no doubt find it helpful to record some of these items on the patient's chart so that you can refer to the chart quickly as the patient enters, and thereby recall a few main points of interest about him or her. Frequently these notations need only be recorded as a single word, such as "golf," "fishes," "sews," "swimmer," and the like. It then becomes an easy task to recall previous conversations with Mrs. Jones about her latest creative work of sewing, or Mr. Smith about breaking par the other day.

Points on Keeping Your Patients Happy

In continuing this same line of thought, once you have established your "happy" patients, it certainly behooves you to keep these same "happy" patients happy. One of the most common problems found in sick dental practices is complacency. The dentist and staff work very hard for several years in reaching a goal of established dental practice, and then, having "arrived," become complacent. There seems to be an ample supply of patients, and seemingly plenty of new ones coming in. But if, after a while, this doctor and his staff begin to really look at their practice, they gradually begin to realize that they no longer seem to generate the enthusiasm from their patients as they once did. Some of their old standbys have stopped coming in as regularly or at all.

These patients have begun to feel that the office is neglecting them. They feel that they are being taken for granted, and no person likes to feel this way. The attitude frequently becomes, "If they no longer care about me (or my business), then I'll just go to someone who does."

This problem seems to be a particularly difficult one if the dentist has previously put the patient through a massive rehabilitation program, and now there is very little dentistry left to do. It easily becomes the attitude of the patient that now that all of this major work has been done and he has spent a large sum of money, and there is little left to do, he is now relegated to the "*minor*" recall list, with the entire staff losing interest in him. How many times have you seen this happen in *your* office?

Let me tell you this—this patient has devoted a great deal of time, energy, money—perhaps the figurative "blood, sweat, tears," and has devoted himself to your office and its principles. He became "dedicated" to permitting you and your colleagues to treat him. You must uphold your end of this dedication by never permitting complacency to enter the picture. This patient has literally paid for your never-ending interest, so do not forget it.

Mr. Jones will always be interested that you wish to know how his family is getting along. Certainly, you ask him each time he comes into the office, but each time he arrives, his children are a little older, and things have changed somewhat.

As you carry patients through the years, children will grow, marry and move away, and this is always a good point to follow. Where are the children? Any grandchildren? Any photographs? It becomes the same old thing of truly being interested in someone and showing it.

It doesn't matter if in reality you detest Mr. Smith. You must always realize he is as important to this dental practice as any patient you have. It has been found that if you will try very hard to understand the viewpoints of someone you dislike, then you may actually find that you don't really find him quite so disagreeable.

How to Keep Your Boss Happy

As has already been noted, the importance of making and keeping happy, enthusiastic patients cannot be overemphasized. The same emphasis must absolutely be placed on the matter of keeping your employer well contented. The key here is his confidence in you. He simply must know at all times—with never any doubt—that you are performing your assigned tasks as you know he wants them performed. He must know that you never permit your own personal problems to interfere with your duties.

Please try hard not to burden your dentist with your personal problems. The doctor has more than enough just taking proper care of his many patients, plus his own family. If you simply must unburden yourself, be absolutely sure it is not during working hours, and the best time would be after work. In this way there will be no need to disturb the doctor's thoughts while he is treating patients, and by the next morning, things may be looking better. Have you thought of this? Why not discuss your problem with the doctor's wife? She certainly has a vested interest in your problems because you work for her husband. She can frequently know the quantity of problems her husband may have at a certain time, and therefore may very well know when it might be best to work with him on your difficulty.

One of the more intriguing ways to keep a boss happy is to surprise him from time to time with something out of the ordinary that you and your associates may do for him. It may be that you will wish to take him out to lunch. In this way you are saying thank you for his being nice to you. You can certainly rest assured that he will bend over backwards trying to return the favor. Don't forget to clear this with the good doctor's wife, however, in order not to offend her.

It sometimes becomes a little boring around a dental office, and so a little spice helps occasionally. What kind of spice? Let your imagination run around for a while. If you type up a daily work schedule, do you think that the dentist and the chairside assistant would like it if you added a short cheerful note or item to it? Then each time they look at it during the day, they will receive a little cheer! What can you say? Anything—"It's Monday, aug-g-gh!" Or, "Friday, Ithoughtit'dnevercome, Jan. 23!" Or, add a humorous line in between all of the rest of the appointed names, such as 9:00, Mrs. Jones; 9:45, Mr. Smith; 10:15, Bobby Black; 10:30, Five-hour rest period; 11:00, Mr. Johnson;. . . etc. You will soon find that the rest of the office staff will look forward to your little surprise notes, and a great deal of cheer will be the result.

You can also place similar notes of cheer in out-of-the-way places (where patients will never see them) that the staff will "find" from time to time. It is little pleasant surprises such as these that help make a long day short.

One obvious point is to keep the dentist informed on the goings-on in the business office. He may not ask you each day what has happened, who has called for appointments, etc., but he certainly should be interested in the high points. Let him know that, "Today, six new patients called and made appointments." "Collections were better than usual today." And, especially tell him things like, "Mrs. Blowhard called today complaining about her bill and I worked it all out with her and now she is happy again."

It is necessary to tell him the bad things that happen too, but you can probably ease these things into his day at some point other than when he has just had a miserable time with a patient. If you can feel or know that he is in a bad mood or has had a bad time, try to find something good to give him with the bad. It just makes things not quite so bad that way. Good dentistry requires great depths of concentration and effort, and a little happiness around the office makes the strain a little less burdensome.

If you really want to keep your boss happy, never, never pry into his personal affairs or phone calls. He will only feel that you are butting in where you have no business. You have been employed to become his "girl Friday" and to work closely with him and to know as much as possible about his wishes and thoughts concerning the business of dentistry, but you must tread very lightly around his other concerns. Always, always take the position that his personal interests are not your concern, and that if he wishes you to know something extracurricular, he will tell you. You will find it in your best interests to show him no encouragement if he seems to want to include you in his personal affairs. Remember, you are only his employee. You will never go wrong if you insist on keeping a strictly employer-employee relationship.

There is one further note that hardly needs to be mentioned to the professional dental auxiliary. As you have spent time around your employer and quite naturally will have unavoidably overheard many of his personal phone calls and conversations, you will learn many facts about his personal affairs. Please accept them as *his* affairs, not yours, and let them go no further. They are as confidential as any information concerning your patients, and there must never be any leak out of the office walls—even to your husband. Even an inkling that some privileged information has been leaked by you can shatter your employer's confidence in you forever.

Never take part in or encourage discussion about the doctor's personal life and affairs with other members of the staff. This would only undermine mutual respect.

Eliminating Confusion in the Business Office

Since the "business of dentistry" begins in the business office, it behooves the smart dental secretary to keep her office at peak efficiency at all times. Any ingress of sloppiness here can only lead to turmoil elsewhere in the dental suite.

As a professional, you are quite certainly aware that there are a myriad of items that you must continually keep track of each day, week, and month. There are the patients to contact continually, the dollars to account for, the telephone calls, the orders from the doctor, the supply lists, the printing, and so on, ad infinitum. It is your task to keep order on all this and still keep from letting things get out of hand.

There are two basic methods of good organization in the business office that will work to eliminate confusion. The first, and most important, is to keep things scheduled. You have an appointment book for the scheduling of the patients, but what I mean is to schedule your own duties. Do this on a daily, weekly, and monthly basis. If you will take an hour or so out some evening, or weekend, you will find it relatively easy to lay out a very complete and simplified plan for each day. Then, as your day goes by, it becomes a simple matter of following your own prearranged schedule for your assigned chores, and do them one by one.

On this chore list or schedule you should have things like: (1) freshen up reception room, (2) post checks after mail arrives, (3) confirm tomorrow's patients, (4) check on postoperative patients, (5) pull tomorrow's charts, etc. You should set out every individual task and list it in the most logical order to insure a smooth, efficient day. No doubt, you will need to alter the schedule after a few days of trial, because of something you may have forgotton to add, but this is no difficult problem. Usually, after one or two weeks, you will have developed a very workable daily schedule. It will undoubtedly be quite surprising to you when you find you have a great deal of time left over during the day. You will have eliminated much wasted motion, and will be quite efficient.

You will need to make up such a schedule for chores that only need to be done weekly, or twice-weekly, and also for the monthly tasks. Make up all of these several lists, and staple them together at the top of the paper, and tack them onto the back of the business office door, or the side of the filing cabinet, or perhaps on the wall, but at least some convenient, out-of-the-way place in the office. Then you can glance at it whenever necessary during your day, and know where you are, and what needs to be done next. It will be only a short time before you have this schedule memorized and will no longer need to refer to it for your aid. It will be helpful to return to it from time to time, however, and review your day against it. In this way you can eliminate missed steps and/or sloppiness before they occur.

You will no doubt find it helpful to inform your doctor of your list, and especially any open spaces you develop in it during the day. This may be the best time for him to dictate letters to you, or have you run errands, or other tasks. It will in this way permit him to work within your efficient schedule whenever possible. He will know that, say, about three o'clock you will have a little time, so he can postpone sending you after some supplies until then, and you will not necessarily have to break into the middle of some posting or typing.

The second vital key to ending confusion is the note pad—just a simple small pad of paper. On this pad—which you keep always at hand—will be written every key word or statement necessary to jog your memory. The doctor is to call someone at two o'clock—write it down. You need to mail some X-rays to another dentist—write it down. You need to order some supplies from the local stationery store—write it down. Now when each item you have recorded has been followed through to its proper completion, you cross it off. When every item on a sheet of paper is crossed off, then, and not before, do you tear it off and throw it away.

Most five-and-dime stores or stationery stores have small two-by-four inch blank paper pads that are economical and handy for this purpose. If you cannot locate any this way, your local printer will usually have some "scratch pads" available, or will make you some. A point here is to use small pads. If you get a size larger than two-by-three or two-by-four, you will waste more sheets, and in addition it will be too bulky to be very handy.

If you can keep away from writing such notes and minor items on the patients' appointment book, you will find that it will be neater, and you can read it more easily and therefore more quickly and efficiently when trying to schedule in a patient. The pads are much better.

How to Properly Accept Delegation

In order to operate a smooth-running, efficient, and productive dental practice, the dentist must of necessity delegate many duties. In fact, if you carry this to its utmost, the only thing the dentist should do in his office is the basic dentistry itself, and absolutely nothing else. This means the auxiliary personnel must handle every other duty, and it is their responsibility to perform these tasks as well as the dentist himself could do it. Therefore this must become your byword: "Am I doing this duty with the skill and dedication that my doctor would use?"

This simply means that for every individual task you perform around the dental office, no matter how simple and trivial it seems to you, you must always place yourself in your employer's shoes. How would *he* do it? Why is it to be done? How much care should I use? Do I have ample skills to do it? If you do not have the proper knowledge and training for a specific duty, then it behooves you to let your doctor know it. It also becomes your duty to learn to do this task as quickly as possible, so that you can relieve him from having to perform it.

Always keep this in mind: the more you can do for him, the more he can do for patients. The more productive he is, it follows that the more he could presumably afford to pay you, doesn't it? So keep your eyes and ears open at all times for new ways to help your doctor. Call for conferences to discuss various aspects of the dental procedures that you might take on for him. Try your best to keep him from performing any task in the office that can be done legally and ethically without a degree in dentistry. The entire organization will be better because of it.

2

Telephone Tips That Will Help You Accomplish More

The Importance of Your Smile

A great deal of time is spent by you, the dental secretary, using the telephone. You receive calls, and you make about as many outgoing calls. Each contact you make with a patient or anyone else is a direct picture of your dental office. You will create an influence upon every person with whom you speak and you know that it must always be a favorable impression that you make. When people talk with you over the telephone, they form their impression on two things: what you say, and how you say it. You can make a declarative sentence actually sound like two different statements simply by changing the emphasis used in the sentence. For example, if you say, "The child *ran* across the street," you have the sentence saying the child probably should have walked across the street. When you say, "The child ran across the *street*," with the emphasis on "street," you may be saying the child should not have run across the street, but should have run across the yard, or field, etc. So it is quite easy to understand why people so frequently misunderstand each other. And remember, your voice sounds somewhat muffled over a telephone.

One of the more interesting aspects of telephone conversation is the fact that one can actually "hear" a smile over a telephone receiver. Try it sometime. Have a friend, or one of your co-workers call you over a telephone. Have them make a simple statement with a frown on their face. Now have them make the same statement with a definite smile on their face, and *you* listen and interpret the difference in the tone and quality of their voice. One hundred percent of the time, the smiling voice will be more pleasant, and smooth. There will be no harshness in the tones.

Therefore, my suggestion is to place a small pocket or hand mirror on the wall beside the telephone or on the desk beside it, where you will be able to watch yourself every time you use the telephone. Now make certain that you create a definite smile habit every time you speak over the phone—to anyone, for any reason. Your patients will notice the difference, and will frequently comment on what a nice telephone voice you have. And what may be surprising to you is that you will somehow get more cooperation from them about things you need to do. It is always much easier to accept someone's viewpoint when they are pleasant, than it is when they are not so pleasant, isn't it?

Another point to remember when using the telephone is to slow down slightly in your speaking speed. Remember, the person is not there in the same room with you, and cannot hear quite as clearly as if he were, so if you will just take a little more time to say what you need to, the listener will be able to understand you more clearly, and will accept you better. This is much easier said than done, however, due to the fact that the dental secretary is frequently quite rushed. Even so, you will find that you will usually save just a little more time when you speak slightly slower, due to the fact that you will not need to repeat yourself in your conversation so much.

How to Satisfy the Angry Patient

One of the most disturbing things in your day will probably happen when you are at your busiest, and you are completely overwhelmed and frustrated at the amount of work you have yet to do, when the angry patient calls you! Now this is a patient who feels he or she has a very legitimate complaint, and is considered by your doctor to be a V.I.P. Somehow you must find a way to soothe the patient, and yet remain in control of the situation enough to settle it equitably for the office.

Step one: Smile! Don't forget, the smile will automatically help to keep you from getting angry yourself, and this is absolutely vital. If you ever find yourself getting angry with a patient with whom you are conversing over the telephone, the only thing for you to do is to excuse yourself, and tell the patient that you will call him right back. Then do return the call, but not until you have completely regained your normal composure. If a patient ever detects anger in you, you have automatically lost the argument.

Step two: Accept everything the patient has to say in as pleasant a voice as possible. It is usually better to say as little as possible, beyond "yes sir" or "no sir." It is important also to let the patient have his say completely. And then, when he seems to be through talking your ear off, politely ask him if there is anything else (that he feels is wrong, or that is bothering him). This will immediately disarm him, and will tend to place him in a defensive position.

Frequently, when he has had his say, and you ask him if anything else is wrong, the patient will tend to backtrack apologetically and will begin to hedge somewhat on the massiveness of the problem. He called to declare war, and found immediately that he was received by a pleasant voice that acknowledged everything he had to say, and then asked for more. He had counted on getting an argument, and you have thrown him off balance. Now all you have to do is either one-by-one answer his objections to the best of your ability, or tell him you will speak to the doctor and call him back about it. This is important: when you tell him you will call him back, give him a specific time limit by which you will call. And make sure you do. If you have told him you will return his call by three o'clock, and you don't, then he can only feel you are ignoring him, and once again you will have an angry patient on your hands. Likewise, if you do not give him some idea about when you will return the call, he will feel a possible brush-off.

Remember this: he feels as though he has a legitimate reason to complain, or he wouldn't call. And he expects satisfaction in one form or another, or he wouldn't call. You must acknowledge his feelings, and accept his ideas of his problem, but not give away basic professional rights of the office or doctor. The professional dignity and standards of the doctor and staff must be upheld at all times and through all forms of harassment. This is your duty. If anyone is to decide that the patient's complaints cannot be relieved, it must be the doctor. If the practice is to lose an angry patient, let it be the doctor's decision, not yours.

How to Handle the "Shopper"

One of the most annoying persons to call you over the telephone is the patient who is obviously just "shopping" around for the cheapest dentist. She is not the least bit interested in quality, but feels only that her dental health can be bought like this week's hamburger.

At this point you can do one of several things, depending on the basic wishes of your dentist.

You can give her a quick brush-off by simply saying you do not quote fees over the telephone. Then there will probably be very little left to say. She will either go ahead and make an appointment, or else she will close the conversation.

Or, you can proceed to tell her whatever fees she wishes to know. There may possibly be no real problem in doing this, provided your dentist has no objections. It is important to remember, however, to point out to the calling party that these fees just might vary from person to person, or from case to case, depending on the exact circumstances. You would certainly not want to give her the idea that one patient might be charged more than another, just because of who that patient might be, or on the whim of your doctor, but rather the variation might come from a case being more difficult, or time-consuming than another.

Probably the best answer you could give a fee-inquiring patient would not be that you do not quote fees over the telephone, but rather that each case can be so widely varied, that it is actually impossible to mention a specific fee without seeing the patient personally. You could, depending on your doctor's wishes, mention casually that while one patient might have a filling costing, say, fifteen dollars, the very next patient might have one similar in size, but requiring more time, or bases, or anesthetics, and end up costing, say, twenty dollars. Or, if you wished, you could project this example downward, to perhaps, ten dollars.

Bear this in mind: it has been shown recently that to quote a fee to a patient, even over the telephone, and sight unseen, actually forms a legal contract that binds the doctor to that specific fee for that specific service. Make quite certain that you never do this to your dentist without his direct permission—not just his implied consent.

Basically, it is generally thought that the best answer to the shopping patient is education of the patient. It is quite impossible to educate the shopper as completely as desirable in a mere minute or two, but this patient must surely realize she is not calling just another ordinary dental office. You must first understand the patient with whom you are speaking. Mr. or Mrs. Jones may actually be very highly educated, perhaps a college professor, or even a physician's wife, but you can quickly assume correctly that he or she is not well educated dentally. It therefore becomes your first goal to pass a word or two to Mr. Jones that he is speaking about something that has much more importance than he realized. You can say something like this: "Mr. Jones, although there are usual and customary fees for specific services around this community, Dr. Blank's philosophy is to serve each and every patient as fairly as possible. He also strives to be as thorough as possible, and therefore feels that he can only offer his best service by way of a complete and thorough examination. After he has performed this service, he will gladly discuss in specific detail all aspects of your necessary dentistry and the related fees with you. The benefit to you will be a total viewpoint of your dental health and a good look into your future needs and necessary outlays. Then you can make a good decision about the kind of dental care you want."

If the patient rejects this advice, you have lost nothing, and the patient will no doubt realize that Dr. Blank is strictly a competent and thorough dentist. When Mr. Jones tires of shopping for the cheapest dentistry around, and finally requires a complete rehabilitation, he will no doubt remember your short comments, and possibly call for an examination with Dr. Blank. You have sown the seeds of dental education for Mr. Jones.

If, however, Mr. Jones decides to accept the time for the complete examination, you have preset his mind to accept the fact that your office practices fair, complete, thorough dentistry, and thereby may be more likely to readily accept Dr. Blank's recommendations.

If you can ascertain that the shopper simply feels as though she needs a single filling replaced, then you can proceed somewhat through your "talk," but then continue that Dr. Blank will gladly treat just a single tooth for her if she so wishes. This will at least get her into the dental office, and then you and the rest of the staff can bring her dental education along as you see fit to do so. In this way, you will have not made a potential patient angry by outright rejection, and you may turn her into a very fine booster for better dentistry.

How to Impress the New Patient

The most common way patients first come in contact with the dental office is by way of the telephone. It is here that first impressions are so very important. The patient who calls and hears a clear, sharp, and cheery voice on the line will undoubtedly be much more respondent than on hearing just another dull, bored, draggy and ho-hum type person on the line. This patient can only assume that this is the type of dentist your doctor is, due to the fact that he hires such a dull person. Think back a moment to a few of your last several telephone calls. Were they all with as fresh and pleasant a voice as you are capable? They should all have that certain something that clearly says you are someone who is first rate.

Remember, each and every telephone call coming into the dental office may be a brand-new patient, curious as to how he will be received and treated. He is curious as to the type of people he will meet here and place his confidence in. From the very first moment of contact with your office, he must know beyond any doubt that he has made the best possible decision, and called the correct office. Almost every patient has some doubts or at least some apprehension when contacting a prospective new dentist. It can be up to you to give him the confidence he needs, or to shatter his aplomb completely.

You must make every attempt to have every patient hang up the phone receiver feeling better than he did when he first called. This you can do simply with enough self-assurance and charm to your voice and conversation. You need not have honey dripping from every word, and you must absolutely learn to be yourself. Any dummy will quickly realize that you are just a put-on, a smoothy. You must *be* self-assured, sharp, charming, cheerful, and above all, helpful. You must be as helpful as you possibly can. You should let this patient know that you are there solely for his bene-fit, and that you have no one else to worry about. He must be made to feel that at this moment, he is the most important patient in your practice, as indeed he may very well be! If you will always remember that, then you will find it quite easy to be the charming and sharp individual that the dentist hired you to be.

How to Start Things Off with Success

Let us assume that your new patient has called, and made a reservation for an initial examination. He probably knows very little about your office or the procedures. He is apprehensive, and somewhat frightened about potential pain or discomfort. Can anything be done to help him? Absolutely!

When you call the day prior to his reservation to confirm and verify the time, you should speak directly to the patient. You certainly tell (remind) him of his time with Dr. Blank, but then you go on. You point out that tomorrow he will be coming in for as complete a dental examination as he has ever had. A thorough history will be taken (by the doctor or one of the staff). Tell him the doctor will want to know about any medical disruptions he has had, and if there are any specific medical or dental problems he may be aware of. The doctor will want to know about his home care and habits. So now that the patient knows that you will be investigating him to this degree of thoroughness, he will begin to think of points of information he will need to bring along.

You point out that the doctor will perform a complete oral

examination as well as a dental examination, and will study the tissues of the mouth to insure the absence of hidden tumors or difficulties. The doctor and his assistant will completely chart his mouth, and note all old dental work and its present state of repair, as well as any new difficulties that have occurred.

Finally, the doctor will take impressions of the upper and lower jaws ("dental arch" may sound too technical for most patients), so he can better study the teeth, and then a complete series of X-rays (radiographs, if your doctor prefers) will be taken.

All of this should take no more than forty-five minutes, and should be completely without discomfort.

Now, what have you said and done? You have properly prepared the patient for everything the doctor may wish to do, so there will be no last-minute objections or particular interruptions. You have planted the idea of thoroughness and completeness into the patient's mind, and you can well believe he is going to be thinking of that dental appointment with considerable interest and anticipation because of his eagerness to see all of this complex diagnostic examination take place. An awful lot of effort is going to be spent on him tomorrow—just for him! He is in the center ring. He is Mister Big.

You have let him know about how much time he will need to reserve away from his normal activities. He now knows to expect no pain.

He must also think about his home care, and will quite likely have his teeth and mouth somewhat cleaner for the doctor than usual.

In short, Mr. Patient has had most of his fears and apprehensions soothed prior to the appointment, and he will be a much better, and a more appreciative patient because of it.

3

Developing an Effective Appointment Book

It All Starts Here

How many times have you said to yourself, "Oh, that blankety-blank appointment book!"? Or, "I'm going nutty because of that appointment book." Or, "I've a good mind to throw that darn thing right out the window!" Certainly an ill-controlled appointment book can create more havoc and disruption in a dental office than anything else. After all, it is a written pattern of your entire week. Everything done in the dental office—every simple task or chore—is either directly or indirectly related to what is found here. If there are no patients, there will be no dental practice. If you have had a frenzied week, a glance back at the schedule will show you why. If you had an easy, smooth-running week, again a backward glance will clearly show you why.

Next Monday before work ask yourself what kind of week we had last week. Then get out last week's appointment schedule and have yourself a big laugh. This should help you start your week off on a cheerful note! Did that really happen to us? Or perhaps you should say to yourself, "How could I have possibly done that to my doctor?'' Or–did your doctor do that to you? Mutual? Isn't that an interesting thought?

The key to the successful dental practice and the so-called well-oiled machine is right here–the appointment book. And you've heard this for years in lectures as well as in the literature. The point is that you must make the decision now–henceforth to control "the book"–not to let it control you. (Isn't it actually the patients who are controlling it?) It is not in anyone's best interest to be like a fallen leaf–just floating along in the breeze–yielding to any slight pressure from any direction. It is solely up to you to stand strong, and to make certain basic rules and plans for the appointment book and to follow through with them. This will create peace of mind for you and the entire office.

How to Control the Appointment Book

Now that you have made your decision to correct the situation with the cluttered, disorganized appointment book, there are certain necessary steps to follow:

First, before moving any further, you must have a talk with your doctor. Tell him what your thoughts are and why you feel a correction is in order. It will be necessary to convince him the "AB" (appointment book) will produce more income for the office, while at the same time, render an easier, more comfortable and therefore, a more enjoyable day. If there is any doubt in his mind that this can be made to happen, then you better not make any major changes. Each doctor has his own particular feeling of security, and your doctor may feel more comfortable leaving things as they are. I would suggest, however, that you at least plant the seed in his mind of a change for the better and thus you may eventually see a better situation evolve. After you have his permission, the next step is to follow through. Here is what to do:

Set aside your next afternoon off, or a Saturday morning. Make every attempt to get the entire staff present–especially the doctor.

Now, you first must skeletonize the AB. This means to completely remove all names and appointments from it. Of course, in order to preserve your sanity, it might be best to simply start with a new, blank appointment schedule. If you use a loose-leaf system, so much the better, but otherwise, a new book will be the simpler way out.

As you remove each name from the AB, record it, and the length of time allotted, and also note if any other appointments are scheduled for the same individual.

At this point the doctor must make a decision about his method of practicing. He can either use numerous short appointments (say thirty minutes each) or else he can combine patients' appointments into longer, but fewer appointments. It may be pointed out here that the shorter appointments give the doctor and the staff more frequent breaks during the day, as they move from patient to patient, and usually, the patient does not receive a particularly large fee each time.

On the other hand, the longer appointments permit more efficiency and reduce overhead for the office, and a larger production schedule is permitted daily. Your patients' paying habits may need to be altered accordingly, as noted in a later section of this chapter.

Anyway, once the decision has been made, then you can proceed to the AB and now block out times for various lengths of appointments. Put no names in now! The longer blocks of time should be set up first, then fill in the shorter ones around them. Your daily sheet may thus look similar to the example shown in Figure 3-1.

In this example of a typical week in the appointment book, the dental secretary has preset appointments for both the doctor and the hygienist. She has set up a number of longer times scattered variously throughout the week in order to give patients some opportunity to fit their own schedules into this. A few short appointments are set out each day as anticipated a week or so in advance, in order to do those single occlusals or suture removals or dressing changes.

These preset time slots can readily be altered a week or so in advance if it is seen that Mrs. Gotrocks will be coming in for treatment soon and will need several extra-length reservations. Also, if needed, the longer times can be reduced to multiple short ones easily.

Note also that the hygienist has a number of varied-length time slots set up so she can more efficiently see adults and children at specific times. She may desire a full hour on Mr. Pipesmoker, so the secretary can easily convert the three-quarter time at four o'clock on Monday, January 2, into a full hour, by eliminating the 4:45 time slot. Or, if preferred by the hygienist, she can keep the quarter-hour slot for a follow-up appointment for plaque control. It will be seen that she plans to spend most of her time on Tuesday afternoon working on children, with half-hour appointments. Likewise, the doctor will be seeing several patients also, so will likely have a fairly easy time breaking out of his schedule frequently in order to check the hygienist's patients.

You will note the preset longer appointments are 9-10:30, 10:45-12:00, 2-3:30, and the remaining times are various lengths of shorter times. Of course, any variety of spacing may be used for the longer appointments—suitable for the doctor.

Emergency time for this schedule can be easily set aside at 10:30 or 12:30. If you wish an afternoon emergency time, you can move lunch hour from 12:45 to 1:45, and have an opening at 3:15.

It is suggested that you look back at the schedule over the past year and more or less average the number of emergency patients your doctor's practice carries. In this way you can have a good idea as to how to better set aside the emergency time in advance without having it go by as free, unfilled time. You may be able to know fairly accurately, for instance, that you will have more emergencies than normal during January and August, (or some other particular month). Thereby you can set aside two emergency times daily for these months, or one longer one, etc. The rest of the year, you may find one fifteen-minute appointment daily sufficient to carry the emergency load. Naturally, emergencies can never be accurately planned for, but "guesstimates" will help.

Where there are fairly infrequent emergencies, say two to three times weekly, it may help to set aside one hour and fifteen minutes for lunch. Any emergency can then be seen just prior to lunch (or just after) and if none come in, the doctor and the staff get a more leisurely luncheon.

This extra fifteen minutes is also an excellent time for staff meetings, or if the doctor so desires, he can readily use the time for X-ray reading and case planning.

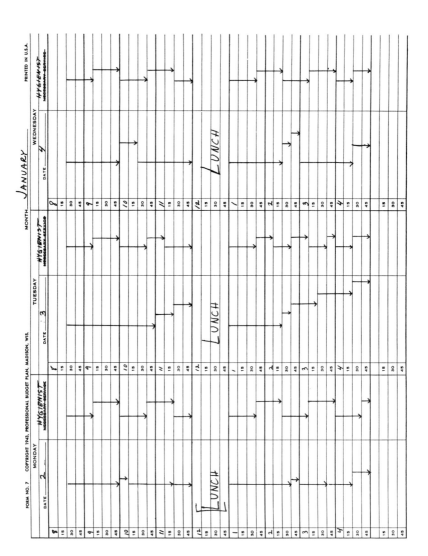

Figure 3-1: Appointment Book

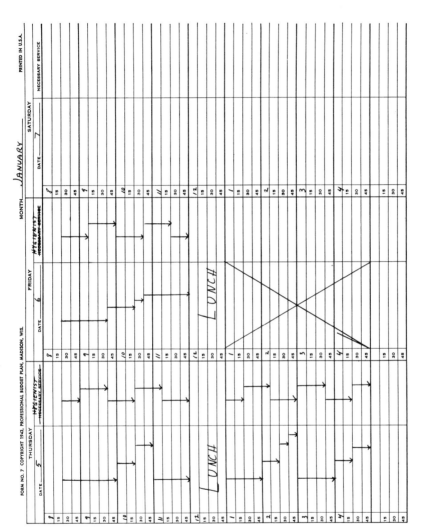

Figure 3-1: Appointment Book

If the doctor likes short appointments, at least try to prearrange the schedule so that he performs different services at alternate times. This will permit more variety, and thereby, less boredom. (This will also permit full sterilizer time between patients if the same instrument is needed for two separate patients. There will be less likelihood of inadequate sterilization if the chairside assistant can leave them in the sterilizer while an alternate procedure is being performed.) Your schedule may thus run something like this: operative, periodontia, prosthetics, operative, crown and bridge, operative, endodontia, periodontia, and so forth, instead of operative, operative, operative, periodontia, periodontia, endodontia, and so on.

Always keep a close eye on the way the AB is moving. If you find you need longer appointments, you must be able to set them up in advance, and likewise for the shorter ones.

If you can get your dentist to let you, then by all means limit the scheduling of appointments to something in the neighborhood of two weeks maximum. This way you can easily increase the number of longer reservations without seriously affecting any patient's time. You will find it easy to add emergency time in this same fashion if you expect it to increase (again by using last year as your guide).

An additional advantage of limited appointments is so the doctor can get started right away on Mrs. Gotrocks' $4,000 cash-advance case without the necessity of waiting eight to ten weeks.

Other Forms and Schedules

In the sample work schedule in Figure 3-2 (available from Professional Budget Plan), John Jones prefers Tuesdays and Thursdays for his appointments, so every reasonable effort will be made by the secretary to fit his dental reservations into his preferred schedule.

The dentist will need two hours to prepare the teeth and take impressions on Mr. Jones' left side (upper and lower), and after placing temporaries, will need at least fourteen days for laboratory construction time before his next appointment.

The second appointment will involve the placement of the castings, and then the preparation and impressions of his right

WORK SCHEDULE FOR _John Jones_

TIME PREFERRED _Tuesdays and Fridays_   DATE _2/1/73_

Time Necessary	Services Planned	Date & Time Appointed		Services Not Completed	Time Necessary
2	Left side preps & impressions				
	allow 14 days				
2 1/4	Seat left side and Right side preps & impressions				
	allow 10 days				
1 1/4	Seat right side and silicates				
1	Prophylaxis & plaque control				
	Recall 4 months				

Figure 3-2: Work Schedule

side. This will require about two and a quarter hours and this time will need only ten days laboratory time.

The final operative appointment will last one and one-quarter hours and will involve the seating of castings on Mr. Jones' right side, plus several silicates.

Finally the patient will receive a final prophylaxis and instruction in plaque control. This can be at the same appointment following the dentist's time, or can be scheduled at a later time a day or so later.

By noting the anticipated time before recall on the work schedule, both the dental hygienist and the secretary can know this without further conversation needed by the doctor.

Name										
¼	½	3/4	①	1¼	1½	1	3/4	2	2¼	2½
¼	½	(3/4)	1	1¼	1½	1	3/4	2	2¼	2½
¼	½	(3/4)	1	1¼	1½	1	3/4	2	2¼	2½

		Days Between:								
Fillings	I									
Prophy	3	2	4	6	⑦	8	10	12	14	16	18
Extraction		2	4	6	⑦	8	10	12	14	16	18
Surgery		2	4	6	7	8	10	12	14	16	18
P&I	I									
Seat	2									
Try-In										
Post-Op										
Impressions										

15

Figure 3-3:   Work Schedule—Short Form

For the appointment such as recalls and where a short chariside case presentation has taken place, it is frequently quicker to have a short-form work schedule. Here it is only necessary to make a very few quick circles or numbers, and it is completed.

In Figure 3-3, routine appointment lengths are set out, then a list of the most-frequently-used operations is made. Under the "Days Between" section are commonly needed numbers. The secretary knows that if no "Days Between" number is circled, the patient can be brought back the very next day.

The blocks to the immediate right of the treatment list give space for the numerical order of the appointments, for example, first, second, and third.

In the example in Figure 3-3, the first appointment needs to be for one hour for P&I (preparation and impressions). Fillings may indicate amalgams or silicates, and may also be done during the P&I time with no further notation needed. If the doctor wishes, however, he can also make a "1" following "fillings," also indicating both fillings and P&I to be done at this time.

The "7" is circled on the first row of the "Days Between" column indicating to the appointment secretary that a week is needed between the first and second trips by the patient to the office.

The second visit will be for three-quarters of an hour for "seating" (and cementation) of the casting.

The final or third appointment will be for a prophylaxis and since no "Days Between" figure is circled, can be on the same date as the "seat" appointment, or any date thereafter.

This brief, simple form has proven to be very efficient and a great time-saver. It can be simply typed out on the office typewriter with multiple carbons, or be printed locally.

If you wish to do so in your office, you can also add a box at the bottom of the slip beneath the "Days Between" section. Into this spot is noted the fee that was due for the work done today by the dentist or hygienist. The chairside assistant gives the work slip to the patient requesting that it be carried to the desk and presented to the appointment secretary.

The secretary then schedules all of the visits necessary and tells the patient the fee for today, so she can (hopefully) accept payment. This way there is no rushing around for a chart to see what was done and how much fee is involved.

How to Make the Appointment Book Your Friend
Instead of Your Enemy

By putting into use the above-mentioned suggestions, it will quickly become apparent that you have a new dental practice with the same old patients. Now you can take the list of the patients that you removed from the original jumbled schedule and group (with the doctor's help) the appointments. Mrs. Jones had four one-half hour appointments for work that can be done in one and one-half hours. You now call Mrs. Jones and schedule her into a one and one-half hour space. By the way, be certain to let Mrs. Jones know that her time is being lengthened in order to save *her* time and to relieve *her* of the worry of having to think about (and remember) so many different appointments. If she is hesitant to proceed with the one and one-half hour appointment, then you may compromise with two one-hour appointments or one one-hour and a half-hour appointment. At any rate, any time you can reduce the number of visits each patient needs, you're way ahead of the game.

Continue grouping appointments in this manner and schedule a week or two of the long appointments. Next begin to fill in the shorter times. Usually this will offer little difficulty. If you have any problems in finding short (half-hour) appointments, you can always temporarily go back to the condensed, longer appointments and break them up into the shorter ones that you need. Naturally, you will not want to alter any times scheduled with patients already.

The planning of the appointment schedule thus becomes a sort of jigsaw puzzle. You simply take the various pieces and fit them into the best places. You can schedule your doctor heavy one day, light the next; heavy in the morning, light in the afternoon. It can almost become fun. It will become a friend.

Ways to Make It Produce Glorious Results

If you really want to have fun with the AB, use the following techniques:

After you *and the doctor* have decided how to most effectively treat Mrs. Smith, you can generally add up the anticipated fee to be charged her at each visit. For instance, her operative appointments may cost her $85 and $70 respectively for two trips, then $290 for a new partial denture, probably requiring two trips, then finally she will need a prophylaxis and home care instructions, $20. So you can record on paper (the back of the work schedule, maybe?) 1-85, 2-70, 3-145 (one-half the fee for the partial), 4-145 (the balance of the fee for the partial), 5-20.

Do this for every possible patient. It will only require a few moments of your time.

Now, you can see that it is quite easy and a great deal of fun to simply add up tomorrow's anticipated production, by noting each of tomorrow's scheduled patients, how much you anticipate their fee will be, and then the total. You will, of course, have a few unknowns along the way as well as a few unavoidable variables, but you will be pleasantly surprised at how accurate you can become. You may even do this same procedure for the next two weeks.

It can become an exciting and interesting contest within the office to see if the doctor and the chairside assistant can top what you have told them to expect!

By utilizing this same method, it is no great problem to schedule in a financially very rewarding day when expecially desired. You simply place into the schedule those patients requiring work that will produce the greatest fees. You can aim for record achievement days and bask in the glory of knowing you and the office produced a $1,000 day! I should not need to point out that you will not want to postpone serious problems or patients with deep decay.

Now, of course, you must not expect to do this every day, because there is always the patient who simply needs a small occlusal amalgam. Sooner or later you have to do this service, too. But these become the good fill-in appointments. Sometimes the numbers of these types of appointments get to be overwhelming. This becomes a good time to schedule in a "junk day." On this day plan no long appointments. Plan no heavy work load in the business office. If you must see twenty patients that day, the staff will certainly have no time for running the bills, or calling this month's recalls, or catching up on back letters. Base the entire day on the premise that everyone will be overloaded simply by the volume of patients, and you will find that the day will slip by much more smoothly than if you had attempted anything else that day.

Some offices schedule a junk day once a week or every other week, or just a half-day every week or so. Make your own decision based on the volume in your office.

Quite frequently, after taking several weeks of patients off the appointment book and rescheduling them, you'll find you have some patients left over—although not as many as you thought you had. You still must not book beyond ten days to two weeks, so what do you do with the leftovers?

Point number one, have the doctor ascertain which patients can be safely postponed and which cannot. Postponing a known near-exposure could be disastrous. Place the leftovers on the call list.

Patient	Telephone	Service Needed	Time Needed	Results
Abrahamson, Dr. J.	765-4321	P&I	3/4	scheduled
Winkler, S.	432-1765	silicates	1¼	
Smithee, Johnny	234-5671	Px, Fl.	1	TCB
Henri, Jacques	123-7654	amals	½	
Thompson, Geo.	135-2468	amals	3/4	
Reed, K.	543-7654	P&I	1½	Mondays only TCB
Ardenne, L.	234-6354	Bridge, seat	1	scheduled
Baker, I. O.	498-6784	FU imps.	3/4	
Carommes, L.	942-5371	try-ins	½	PMs
Henkle, P.	888-2165	px	3/4	

Figure 3-4:   Patient Call List

For this call list, you should have the information listed as in Figure 3-4. After the patient's name and phone number, you need the service to be done, and the time needed. Under the "Results" column you record: "scheduled," or "declined," or "TCB" (To Call Back—this indicates they will call you back later). In this way you will also have a record of what happened when they complained that your office did not take care of the work they needed.

Place a check in the "Results" column every time you call and get a busy signal, and a cross every time you call and receive no answer. This will show you later how much effort you have put into trying to contact this patient.

You must, of course, carefully and confidently explain to Mrs. Johnson that we are rearranging the appointment scheduling so as to be able to treat each patient without the rushed feeling we've had in the past. The doctor feels he can offer a better service to everyone through this rescheduling. Since we felt she would appreciate the doctor's desire to serve better, we want to place her name on our call list for the next available appointment. It should be within the next few days. If she has any trouble or problems have developed, call us back right away and we will see her at our emergency time. Thank her sincerely for her cooperation. If she will not cooperate, we'll change another patient and call Mrs. Johnson back and make an appointment for her. This may require a little "tongue-in-cheek" getting started, but it usually proves successful.

Occasionally a patient will disagree with the change and leave the practice, but if the DA has performed well on the telephone, this is certainly minimized.

On Fitting That Extra Patient into the Busy Schedule

There is always that rather frequent occurrence in every practice where all of your schedule is filled in, including your emergency time, and that patient calls who simply must be seen today. There is absolutely no way to put this patient off, so what to do?

This is where the true professional dental assistant proves that she is worth her salt. You simply must know where the doctor can take a break from his scheduled patients. In order to know this—and you shouldn't interrupt him if you can avoid it—you must know what he is planning to do on each patient, and how he is progressing with the patient in the chair at this time.

You should take a few moments at the beginning of the day to survey the planned work on the scheduled patients as shown in Figure 3-5. This will give you some clues. The doctor will (or will not) give an anesthetic to Patient 1, so he will (or will not) have three or four minutes available to see Patient 2 during the time of patient 1's anesthetic waiting period. Then, he will have a few minutes while the cement on Patient 4's inlay is setting. Or the impression material is setting. Or the chairside assistant is taking X-rays. Or waiting for the development of X-rays for a wet reading.

If you pay close attention to all of these types of details during the working day, you'll no doubt find more than a few opportunities to sneak in that mandatory work-in.

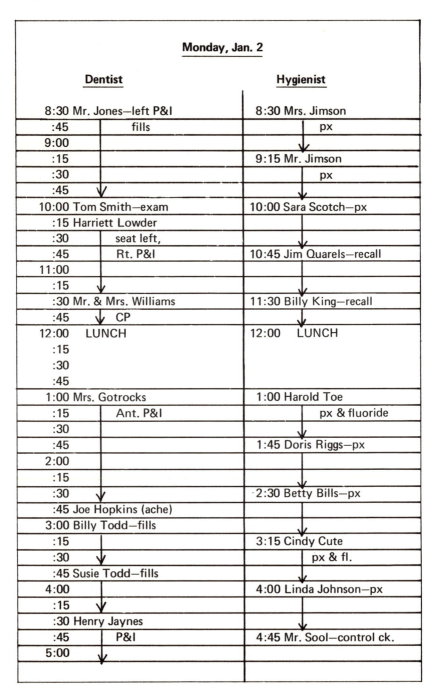

Monday, Jan. 2			
Dentist		**Hygienist**	
8:30 Mr. Jones—left P&I		8:30 Mrs. Jimson	
:45	fills		px
9:00			↓
:15		9:15 Mr. Jimson	
:30			px
:45	↓		↓
10:00 Tom Smith—exam		10:00 Sara Scotch—px	
:15 Harriett Lowder			
:30	seat left,		↓
:45	Rt. P&I	10:45 Jim Quarels—recall	
11:00			
:15	↓		↓
:30 Mr. & Mrs. Williams		11:30 Billy King—recall	
:45	↓ CP		↓
12:00 LUNCH		12:00 LUNCH	
:15			
:30			
:45			
1:00 Mrs. Gotrocks		1:00 Harold Toe	
:15	Ant. P&I		px & fluoride
:30			↓
:45		1:45 Doris Riggs—px	
2:00			
:15			↓
:30	↓	·2:30 Betty Bills—px	
:45 Joe Hopkins (ache)			
3:00 Billy Todd—fills			
:15		3:15 Cindy Cute	
:30	↓		px & fl.
:45 Susie Todd—fills			↓
4:00		4:00 Linda Johnson—px	
:15	↓		
:30 Henry Jaynes			↓
:45	P&I	4:45 Mr. Sool—control ck.	
5:00	↓		

Figure 3-5:   Daily Work Sheet

Actually, if you come right down to it, if you wish to do so (check with the dentist first), you can frequently add a full patient or two to the already filled schedule in this manner. The doctor can anesthetize Patient 1, and while waiting for him to become numb, can go to room two and inject Patient 2. Then he can make the cavity preparation on Patient 1 while Patient 2 is getting numb. Then, while the impression is setting up on Patient 1, the doctor can make the preparation on Patient 2, and so on. As the impression material sets up on Patient 2, the doctor can inject the anesthetic into Patient 3 and then return to Patient 1 for the final checkout and discharge. As you can see, with proper scheduling, this can go on and on.

It certainly must be pointed out, however, that the dentist will have very little time for conversation with either of these patients, and you had better explain to them individually that the doctor is working at peak dental efficiency—not rushing—in order to do them both a favor by treating them today and not making them wait. Don't make the doctor explain—it's better coming from you.

A day like this will obviously be a day of sheer production. The doctor will have little or no time for establishing rapport with his patients, or for making them relaxed or be at ease. Do not start new patients in this fashion! Make absolutely certain all of the auxiliary personnel of the office carry as much of the patient rapport for the doctor as possible. The patient can easily feel he is in an assembly line where no one cares about his feelings, and that the office is only interested in getting the job done and moving on to the next patient. The patient will frequently come to feel that your office is only interested in his money and not his welfare. This can never be permitted to happen. On these rapid-fire days, it will be strictly up to you—the auxiliary—to keep cool, calm, and collected, and to insure that the patients are treated graciously, and in a very friendly fashion when they are there. This is certainly the day when you must pile on the extras. If the doctor cannot remain with the patient at long intervals, then you must try to fill in the void by being there yourself. If this is in turn impossible, at least try to leave the patient some interesting literature to occupy his time.

How to Handle the Habitually Late Patient

Nothing can ruin a finely tuned day more than the late patient, and nothing can disturb a smooth practice like the patient who is *always* late. Sure she has an excuse—she always does. (So do male patients!) The point is, the patient is more interested in other things than her dental appointment.

The secret: Educate this patient to the point where she cares more about the dental appointment—at least where she appreciates its value—than her other interests. Work on her every time she comes in. Tell her all about the wondrous advantages of fine dental work—such as the doctor produces, and how the doctor can do so much for her—not just for now, but for the protection of her health and comfort for the rest of her life. Give her reams of dental literature.

Make up a special folder just for her, and give it to her when she comes in next. You may even make it up while she is in the chair. Have in it reprints and other printed matter pertaining not just to any immediate problems she may have, but also to any other facets of dentistry. Endodontia? Who knows, she may need a root canal some day.

But this education and appreciation process takes time. It is not fair to the doctor or the other patients for one patient to continually throw the schedule off, so try this: schedule her for fifteen minutes prior to the time when you actually want her. If, say, you want her at 3:30, then put her name down in the AB for 3:30—don't let her see this recording—but put on her card 3:15, and tell her 3:15.

Make a note on the AB, "SE." This will remind you when you call next time to remind her of her appointment, that she is *S*cheduled *E*arly, so you will not forget and tell her 3:30 by mistake. That might ruin all your plans.

In your education process, be sure to find an opportunity to have a pleasant, but frank talk with her. Don't make the doctor do it. Point out to her that the doctor has a very busy schedule seeing all the patients that he can that *need* and *want* to be seen. He simply has no extra minutes in the day to waste waiting for someone who is late. If he has to perform certain duties on this patient that take a certain length of time, then he will probably run over into someone else's time, and this isn't fair to anyone. The doctor will never jeopardize his quality by rushing. If the patient arrives so late the doctor cannot see him, then it is wasted time—not only for the doctor, but it also prevented someone else from coming in who perhaps needed to very badly. Yet, by having the time scheduled for him, thinking he would be there, no one else could be scheduled.

The Appointment Breaker

Here is another evildoer. Mrs. Jones with the $4,000 case, *and* a personal friend of the doctor's wife, seems to think nothing of breaking her appointments. And it's not the short, minor appointments she seems to break time after time. She makes the "prophy" appointment, but breaks the two-hour times. And the very next day she calls and apologizes in a sugary voice. And her excuse was "legitimate." And the doctor fumes.

Your solution can only be to have a heart-to-heart talk with Mrs. Jones. This can be over the phone, but you will have far better results if you can speak to her "across a cup of coffee" in your office.

You must, in your most polite and sincere voice and attitude, explain your point of view to her. "Mrs. Jones, this is our problem: we have set up extended appointments specifically for you, at the doctor's request, in order to give him time to perform his very best work for you. He feels it of the utmost importance for your case to be handled in this manner. We have held the work of other patients back especially for you because he feels that you are important. Then when you didn't appear, three things occurred: (1) Your mouth condition deteriorated (even if only so slightly)—this was unfair to you. (2) The doctor had open time—this was unfair to the doctor. (3) Other patients that badly needed to come in could not, because we had reserved that time for you—unfair to them. Now Mrs. Jones, what are your thoughts on all of this? Can you understand our point of view?"

At this point Mrs. Jones is now placed into the position of having to explain her viewpoint in a defensive manner. She will now realize that henceforth any consideration of breaking an appointment on her part will require much more than just a casual thoughtless excuse. She knows she will have some tall explaining to do.

You may point out to her that you realize, of course, that unexpected emergencies do arise, but not every week (we hope).

You may wish to add to your conversation that when you asked the doctor whether or not you should make the *usual charge* for Mrs. Jones' broken appointment, he said *not this time*, but that you'd hate to have to ask him again.

You must certainly ascertain as to whether or not a more convenient time can be set up for her—one she is less likely to find cause to break.

If you have reason to assume that Mrs. Jones is breaking the appointments due to fear of the potential discomfort, then naturally you can point out that many times the doctor prescribes *mild relaxants* to ease any tension or apprehension toward the coming appointment. "Why, we had one patient who was so afraid of her dental appointments, she would become sick just prior to her visits and actually broke several appointments. Finally, we talked with her—just like you and I are doing right now—and we found out why she broke so many. Our doctor prescribed this preappointment medication, and *all* of her remaining appointments have been a breeze. Would you like me to ask the doctor for something for you?"

A major cause for the broken appointment is the lack of ability or the lack of desire of the patient to pay for that visit. He comes in for (and pays for) the short, small fee appointments, but breaks the long ones. Or, he comes for the appointments that are set up just after payday, but breaks the ones at the end of the month.

The key here is to first determine how much his bill will be in total, then determine how many appointments he will need, and set it up so that he will pay (and make sure you tell him) an equal amount each time. Next, set all of his appointments immediately following payday. This may spread his work out over several months, but you will go far toward eliminating the unproductive broken appointment.

You will probably not really know the habits of the new

patient, but you'll certainly be able to control him for all time thereafter.

Actually, the equal-payment-per-appointment is always a good idea for the pay-per-appointment type patient. You will never go wrong. You will be controlling the patient, instead of the patient trying to dictate. Also, his needed dentistry will proceed on a planned schedule, giving him better service. In addition, if the doctor has some extra time on a particular day (due to another broken appointment), he may choose to continue to work on this patient and produce more without fear of the patient getting upset because he produced more than the patient planned to pay.

To repeat for emphasis—always make sure the patient knows he is expected to pay an equal amount per appointment. Occasionally you may get some minor complaint from a patient about this method, so then you can point out that it is *now* the general office policy, which permits all patients to be treated equally and fairly, and that it is the same total fee and the same number of appointments for this individual patient, but that it permits the office to budget its time and finances more evenly and efficiently. This in turn enables the doctor to better operate the business of dentistry, which in turn keeps the fees lower.

4 | *The Recall System and How to Use It*

The Importance of Control Here

One of the basic "bread-and-butter" services around the dental office is built around the recall system. This is the actual keystone of every dental practice, and can truly make or break a dental practice. The lack of enough patients returning on a regular basis can cause great variations in the production of a specific practice such as having sufficient work during any slack periods during the year. On the other hand, having too many recall patients can create such a "log jam" that new patients have difficulty entering the practice. This latter practice could soon burn itself out, and the dentist might have to move his office elsewhere. Certainly you would want neither of these extremes to appear in your doctor's practice.

The key is control and it is basically up to the dental secretary to enforce this control, and to reap the golden harvest of the recall system to its utmost. It does not really matter how old the practice is that you are now working with, as long as you can get the proper system functioning as it should. If you feel there is room for improvement, then call for an office conference with your dentist and both of you sit down and work together for a better system. The ideal: just enough patients to keep the doctor steadily busy, and not so many that there is no spare time in which to see new patients. When I speak of the doctor, I also mean keeping the dental hygienist busy if there is one employed in your office. You do not want to get to the point where the dental hygienist is booked so far in advance that a new patient needing a prophylaxis cannot get onto her schedule for four or five or six months. This would be ridiculous, of course, and would actually lead to poor dentistry by the office, and eventual stagnation of the practice due to dissatisfied patients. This stagnation, incidentally, is when the practice gets so bogged down in vast quantity of patients being on recall so that there is very little room for new patients, and pretty soon the doctor finds that he is finding nothing much new to do on his patients (if he is attempting to do fine dentistry), and he reaches a peak gross income, and can climb no further. His old faithful recall system has him chained and bogged down—stagnant. This drag on a practice can kill the practice as well as the man just as surely as the practice that has too few patients, and is no doubt more dangerous because it creeps up on you slowly, insidiously until you reach a point where you are completely in its grip. Then you have a very busy dental practice that grinds slowly into the mire.

How to Set Up the Best System

You must begin by determining just exactly what problems you have at present in your system. Do you have too many recall patients for the dental hygienist to handle? Too many for your dentist? Too few? Rushed periods? Slack times? Broken appointments? Excessive rescheduling? These are the main difficulties that you are likely to encounter over the years. So again, sit down with your employer and discuss with him the various problems as you see them for his practice, and get his views about his practice. Then you both can consider meeting on common ground. Your idea of too many patients may not be suitable for him, as he may desire a more rushed schedule than you. On the other hand, he may feel like working a somewhat slower pace than he presently has to carry. At any rate, both of you will need to sit down and mutually (his preferences come first, remember) decide exactly what you expect and desire from your recalls. Then you can begin to make the necessary changes toward the better system. As always, change nothing without his definite say-so. And don't forget to include the dental hygienist in on your planned changes—she has a vital role in the practice, too.

What to Do When You Have Too Many Recalls

If your doctor's practice has blossomed into one with excessive patients needing to come in, you have an excellent opportunity to upgrade the practice to a higher level. By this I mean that you can now pick and choose your patients if you or your doctor desire to do so. Your doctor or the hygienist or you can look over the list of recall patients needing to come in at the beginning of each month. You pick out your favorite patients and delete your most disliked ones.

It becomes an interesting dilemma in determining on which level to pick. Should you keep those patients that will pay best? Or those that need your doctor's services most? Or rather those whose personalities fit yours best? This all becomes a personal decision for the doctor, of course.

Many dental offices have classified these patients into basic groupings. These go something like this: Group A—they pay well and appreciate your work (they follow home-care instructions well); Group B—pay well but are lazy with their home care; Group C—pay poorly, but do follow your instructions very well; and Group D—are not interested in your help and do not pay well at all. Most certainly you will want to drop all of your Group D patients from your recall list. It is a real tribute to your office that you have impressed these latter patients sufficiently that they come back on recall at all.

Of course, you keep all the Group A patients. They have become your real "VIPs" in that they become a major referral service for you. On the contrary, you must always be on your guard with these fine patients in order to maintain the excellent rapport you have established with them.

Now your doctor and the hygienist must confer on the

Group B and C patients. It may be that your doctor will want to "load" the recall system with Group B's on certain months when he needs the money a little more, and try to move them to Group A's by more office emphasis on the results of good home care. On the other hand, it is always good for your dentist's ego to work on appreciative patients. Remember, you can always try to upgrade the dental education and aptitude of your Group B patients, but you can rarely improve their paying habits. The methods of upgrading their enthusiasm for home care will be discussed further in chapter 16.

So your basic rule here is to recall only those patients that you desire to recall. Just do not call or send notices or reminders to the others. Some patients may realize that you have neglected them and become offended and leave the practice. Remember, these are patients you do not want anyway.

Some patients will realize you have not recalled them and call for appointments. These you will probably want to see, since they have indicated enough interest to want to come back. If you have classified them as Group B patients, then they are about ready to move up to Group A with only a little help from you. If they are Group C patients, then you can announce to them that your new office policy is strictly cash per appointment. Then they will automatically become Group B patients.

If any "D" patients call, you can make appointments with them if you so desire, but you may wish (with your dentist's permission) to tell them that the practice is closed to any more appointments now. You should suggest that they contact some other dentist. If they should happen to insist, then again you can assume that they are beginning to move upward to a Group B or C level. Then you will be happy to accept them back into the dental practice. If you wish to "save face," you can tell them that you will call them if an appointment opens up, then call them in a couple of days and make the appointment.

What to Do When You Have Too Few Recalls

If your office has too few recalls to keep your doctor or the hygienist busy on any type of reasonable schedule, there must be at least one of three basic problems. You are with a very new dental practice that has not yet had time to accumulate patients. Or perhaps your community is so transient that your patients simply do not stay around long enough to be recalled in any volume. Both of the above difficulties are uncontrollable. A third reason exists—one that can get quite touchy—your patients simply do not care to return. (This assumes, of course, that you do try to contact all potential recall patients.) If you continually sent out recall cards or calls and do not get affirmative results from the vast majority of the patients, then your office is failing somewhere. You must discover what is wrong. It may well be best to take a good close look at your office and see if you can decide why patients might not want to come back. Are there any obvious technical reasons? Is your office dirty? Unkempt? Out of touch? Old-fashioned? Is parking difficult? Poor access?

Or is the problem (in your personal opinion) more one of the way patients are handled while in the office? This is where you may have a very sensitive problem—especially if the major fault seems to lie with the dentist himself. If you determine no other reason, I would suggest that you first discuss the situation discreetly with other auxiliaries who work in the office. If there are no others, or perhaps even if there are, you might privately discuss it with a special friend who is an auxiliary in some other office. Perhaps she can mention something that some of your former patients have said about your office when they came to the other office. Let me emphasize that such action must be held in absolute and discreet confidence. No word of this must be allowed to get either to the other dentist or your own.

If you have finally and absolutely determined that the problem lies entirely with the doctor himself, you must make your own personal decision as to whether or not to mention it to him. If you decide not to say anything, then so be it. However, if you do feel the necessity of mentioning the situation to him, then please approach it with great caution and tact. Bear this in mind—if he becomes overly offended or insulted by what you say, then you may need to find another office in which to work.

I would suggest that you make your suggestions just that—suggestions and ideas that you feel may help get a better reaction from your patients. Remember, it is not *you* they are coming to see, and your personality and mannerisms may not fit your dentist at all. You may ask him if, say, he realizes that what he just said to Mrs. Jones might have been misinterpreted by her and he may have offended her. Or that although you are sure that he did not mean it that way, it sounded as though he cut Mrs. Brown short. Or that if the doctor wished you to do so, you would be quite happy to handle all the office financial arrangements, so that he would not have to bother (and seemingly come across to his patients that he was only interested in their money, not their well-being).

In other words, you are telling the dentist what he is doing wrong, but not in exact, blunt, offending words. Let him grasp the idea in his own thoughts and it will seem more like his idea, instead of making it seem as though you are sticking your nose into his business. You are less likely to hurt his feelings and pride or insult him this way.

If you have peaks and valleys when you have first too many recalls, and later, too few, you may equalize the load by running some patients to seven or eight months and some up to five mouths until you are more level, and then you can get back onto a regular six-month schedule. Be sure you check out each patient as much as possible so as to postpone the seven- and eight-monthers safely and not endanger them, and also, the five-monthers should be those who need somewhat closer attention.

5 | *The Importance of Supply Control*

The Importance of Control Here

The business of dentistry is one that is composed of the delivery of a service. In order to meet this delivery obligation properly, needed supplies must be on hand and readily available at all times. Woe unto those responsible when the dentist has already prepared the cavity preparation, and then discovers that he is out of, say, shade eight filling material. No other color will suffice, and Mrs. Prissy just will not be brought back, nor will she accept any other color. Just what is your doctor to do? Borrow some from a nearby dentist? Perhaps. At least he would certainly hope to do so. And, of course, this points out to his colleagues (in an embarrassing manner) that his office is run in such a sloppy fashion that you run out of vital supplies. Now he must not only order more supplies, but he must also remember to order an extra amount with which to pay some back to the other dentist.

The obvious answer is to have such an efficient system set up in your office that such a situation will never occur. You must be able to have sufficient supplies on hand at all times to meet any normal calls, plus an amount in reserve for contingencies or emergencies.

How to Set Up the Best System

In order to get started on a really successful and controlled supply system, you must first know what you have, and what you need. In addition you must discover how much of which materials that you use. This will tell you how frequently you will need to reorder.

The simplest place to begin is in the operatory. It is most frequently here that the majority of the daily-use materials are kept. Just start with pad of paper, and record in the order that you see it, each material as you come to it. Start on the cabinet or counter top, and record each item that might be used up. Next go down into the cabinet into each drawer and likewise record each item found there. When you get to the burs, you will need to note each type specifically. That is, "right angle, ¼, ½, 1, 2, . . . ;" "friction grip, ¼, ½, 1, 2, . . . ;" "straight handpiece burs, steel, ½, 1, 2, . . . ;" "straight handpiece burs, carbide, ½, 1, 2, etc."

After completing all the supplies in one operatory, move to the next one, and make sure there is nothing in this one that you do not already have on the list. Then follow through in each operatory. It will usually follow that even though your doctor may have two "identically equipped" operatories, you can usually find a few minor variations in supplies, and each of these will need to be noted on your list. Don't forget the hygienist's room, and all of her consumables. What about the dark room, and the X-ray film (different speeds, sizes, types), and the developer and fixer concentrates?

Naturally, the next place to go is into the laboratory or wherever your office keeps its main bulk stocks.

Let me point out here that by this time your list is getting rather long and cumbersome. You will also have noted that you are having to spend a fair amount of time on this project. You will find it better to resign yourself to the fact that it is a task better spaced over several days, than to try to jump into it all in one day. Just make sure you complete each location before you stop each time. In other words, do not stop in the middle of a cabinet or especially a drawer if at all possible. You might just find yourself losing your place and duplicating your listing, or worse, skipping some items.

You might also note that at this time, I have not recommended that you make note of any of the amounts of these consumables you have on hand. You will definitely need to know this later, but it will be better to put this off until proper preparations have been made for the figures. This is just a simple listing of all items that are used up in the routine practice of dentistry, not an inventory.

After you have completed your listing of all the dentally oriented items, you should also make note of all of the business office items, such as letterheads, envelopes, carbon paper, etc. Pencils, and pens, and paper clips, too. Your list is now getting really long, but keep going.

Don't forget toilet tissue, hand soap, paper towels, cleaner, and the like.

Later on, you will also want to list each magazine your doctor subscribes to and its expiration date.

Now that you have at last completed your basic and preliminary stock listing, you are ready to move into phase two—the card file.

The card file is the basic unit of the entire supply system. It is here that you can know at any given moment exactly what supplies you have on hand in the office. You can reorder at a moment's notice directly from this card file whatever you are needing, and thus eliminate the necessity of trying to remember what you need until the supply man drops by, or having to record everything on a separate list, only to be misplaced later.

Get your doctor's permission to take a few dollars out of the petty cash drawer, and go to your local five and dime store, or stationery store, and purchase a small, four-by-six inch file box, with about two hundred and fifty cards to fit. It is also helpful to get alphabetized index cards, but this is not really mandatory.

Next go back to your original itemized list of all the various consumables in the office, and begin by recording each separate item on a card. Try to be as explicit as possible, and arrive at the exact and simplest name for each item. It is possible to group sizes under the same card, such as burs, but you will find it somewhat easier for the total picture if you even have a separate card for each type, as well as size.

You will usually want to record the brand name of each item

also, but if your dentist isn't particular about any specific brand, you may leave this section off. It may well be he will specify a certain brand for a few specific items, and not care about the rest.

You will find it helpful to record the type of unit for each one of your consumables; i.e., bottle, can, package, case, etc. You will need to know how the product is usually sold, such as in lots of six, or three, or gross or whatever.

There are a few things that you will not be able to place on the card at the beginning. You will need to contact your supplier about many items, and the normal costs for specific items. You need to know the best number to purchase for the best price. Do not take it for granted that just because you can get burs cheaper by ordering ten thousand, that your doctor will want you to do this. There are certainly practical considerations here, such as the total amount of dollars to be spent on such and such an item, and whether or not it will have shelf life, and, of course, the amount of room you have for storage in your office. To be on the safe side, find out the "best price" of a particular item, and the "practical price," and present both of these to the doctor and let him decide.

You will want to record the name and address of the supplier. Most frequently this will be from one or two local supply houses, but there may very well be many items that you receive from other sources—independent salsesmen, mail-order houses, and the like. If you wish to save some room on each card, you can simply code the supplier into a number or an initial, and have a separate index card in the front of the file box containing the complete name, and address of each supplier. The telephone number of the supply house is also helpful here.

When to Reorder

A very important section is that of when to reorder certain items. In considering this, you must know the approximate time that it will take you to receive the item once it is ordered. If an item is usually quite difficult to obtain, and may take several days or even weeks to reach your office, then you will need to consider this and may wish to keep more than normal on hand. Likewise, it may not be necessary to keep a large stock of the more commonplace and plentiful items available. Remember, too, that if you are ordering from a mail-order house, you must certainly allow more time for delivery due to possible mail delays.

Certainly it will not be possible for you to set up this card system quickly. In fact, it may even take months; but once you do get it operating, many of your pesky problems will be eliminated, and you will find your office much more efficient. A side effect is that your dental supply man will become more appreciative because you will be able to order more quickly, and thus save him time so that he can go along on his rounds.

One thing you must know at all times is how much of a certain item you have on hand. Complete inventory control is imperative if the system is to work at all in your favor. You most probably will need to consult with your employer about how much or how many of such-and-such an item to keep on hand. It would be best, however, if you will at least try to establish such figures as much as possible yourself before taking his time. Make a special indication for any that you have doubts or questions about and then you will have need to take less of his time to help you. After all, you are trying to save his time, too.

Most of the less frequently used items will be easily noted, and you can usually run a smaller inventory. An example might be cans of quick-set plaster. This example, of course, assumes that you do not use this material frequently. If you do, then some other example might be better. For the illustration, let us assume that your office uses quick-set plaster once every month or so. Therefore one twenty-five pound can may well last you a year or two. In this case, you may want to buy a smaller size can, just to keep from having so much on hand. For a can of some material, you should take it when it first comes in and more or less establish a certain amount left in the can at which point you will need to reorder, say, one-fourth of a can. Now take the edge of a plaster spatula or the equivalent, and place it against the can about one-fourth of the way up, and tap it with a hammer or mallet. This will make a small groove in the can. Do this same thing several times, all around the circumference of the can one-fourth of the way up, and now when you get down to this level in the can, you will be able to see the indentations inside the can, and know that it is time to reorder. Many cans come already marked this way, which makes it easy, but the larger ones will need to be grooved. Naturally, you will need to avoid puncturing the sides of the can. If your office uses a larger wall-type dispenser, then you can reorder at the point when the plaster first reaches the level of the front lip. Each type of bulk supply you have in your office (any that you cannot number or count) will need to have a similar indication made on its container. If it is a bottle, you can mark it with a piece of tape one-fourth of the way up, or mark it with a wax crayon or even one of the new nylon-tipped pens. Since the latter two methods may rub off after several months, you will find the tape best for long-term results. Mark all containers in the entire office in a similar fashion.

Flat packages such as a box of letterheads can be marked by having a special piece of colored paper with the word REORDER written on it. Then place this sheet down in the box or drawer where the stationery is normally kept, as far from the bottom sheet as you need to. Check this first: how fast you normally use these letterheads, then call the printer and find out how quickly he can print you some more and get them delivered to you. These two factors will help you determine just how many sheets up from the bottom you should place the special "reorder" sheet. Use this same procedure for all such items in the office.

All other items in the office are items that can be counted numerically. Again you need to know these points: how fast you use this item, and how long delivery requires. Talk to your doctor and establish a minimum number to permit the stock to reach. Now establish the most desirable or optimum number to keep on hand. This is in reality a more important figure. Record this on the supply card for each item, as well as the date you record it. Now each time you use something up, it is to be noted on the card. For instance, let us assume you are counting tubes of light-bodied impression material. You have established that your best practical purchasing number is nine boxes. This becomes your top figure. Then you record each date that you remove a tube from the box, and the fact that the supply is now down by one. This continues until you reach your reorder figure, say, three tubes, and at that point you contact your salesman for your new order of nine tubes. You should make a notation on the supply card something to the effect of "Reordered, 2-4-71, Smith Dental Co." Then when the order arrives, you place the top figure on the card as nine tubes plus whatever you have remaining, and this becomes your new figure. Record the price of the nine tubes on the card. Always tell your doctor if you note an increase in price in the nine tubes.

Thus, a card for, say, Kerr, Light-Bodied Permlastic would look something like the one shown in Figure 5-1.

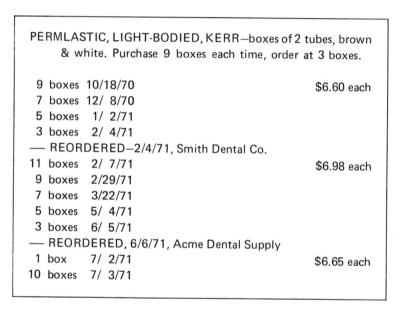

PERMLASTIC, LIGHT-BODIED, KERR—boxes of 2 tubes, brown & white. Purchase 9 boxes each time, order at 3 boxes.

9 boxes	10/18/70	$6.60 each
7 boxes	12/ 8/70	
5 boxes	1/ 2/71	
3 boxes	2/ 4/71	
— REORDERED—2/4/71, Smith Dental Co.		
11 boxes	2/ 7/71	$6.98 each
9 boxes	2/29/71	
7 boxes	3/22/71	
5 boxes	5/ 4/71	
3 boxes	6/ 5/71	
— REORDERED, 6/6/71, Acme Dental Supply		
1 box	7/ 2/71	$6.65 each
10 boxes	7/ 3/71	

Figure 5-1

As you can see from the above illustration, the card would be classified under the main classification of "Permlastic," or under the "P's." Then the subclassification is "light-bodied," and of course, you need the brand name. Should the doctor change brands, but still maintain the same material under a different name, you should switch to a new card. You may save the old card if you wish, but you must make a reference on the new card that there is another card titled "Permlastic." You must also note on the old card to see the new card. Frankly, it is usually rather pointless to save the old card.

If you wish to do so, you may classify all products under type names such as "Rubber base impression material," or such similar titles. However, it has been found that in most offices, the simple one-word description, frequently a widely used brand name is most appropriate.

You can see that the material is being used at the rate of about two tubes every month or so. This would automatically tell you that you go through a tube about every two weeks. So if you get down to a single tube, you have less than two weeks to get a new supply in.

On this simulated card, the material is best bought in batches of nines for the best practical price. At this grouping, the material costs $6.60 per box. When the supply on hand got down to three boxes, more was ordered on that day when the three-box level was reached. A few days grace period in ordering is permissible here because we know from prior experience that Smith Dental Company keeps this material readily available and can supply it for us quickly. It was ordered on February 4, and arrived on February 7. This time its price had gone up from the last price of $6.60 to $6.98. (The price is recorded on a per-unit basis from the invoice enclosed with the package from the supply house.) Your doctor had not yet used up the previous amount of material on hand, so your supply now goes to eleven tubes on hand.

Finally, on June 6, you are once again down to the reorder number of three boxes on hand, so since you have previously pointed out to the doctor that there was a substantial price increase last time, and you have called other local supply houses and noted that they too have similar prices for the material, you searched the mail-order houses, and found one that was only $6.65. So you ordered nine boxes from them.

The in-house supply continues to dwindle, however, until on July 2, you are down to one box. This means you will need some more impression material within a week or so or you will run out. However, on July 3, the new material arrives and you are now back to ten boxes.

At this point you and the dentist must make a decision. You must decide to either pay more per box and keep the reorder at three-box level, and expect prompt delivery, or you will pay the lesser price, up the reorder level to four or five boxes, and accept the slow delivery schedules. This creates interesting decisions sometimes, but it does leave you and your office in full control of your supplies, and not dependent on the outside influences of the various supply houses.

How to Handle the Back Order

One of the most annoying and frustrating things you may run into is the "back order." Here you are with everything running smoothly and efficiently with all supplies coming in on schedule and well-controlled, when all of a sudden you receive that fearsome slip, "We are sorry that the item you have ordered is not in stock. . . . " Now you know that you may have to do something fast. First, look up the card for that particular item and note how much you have on hand. Next note how fast it is being used up, and you make a mental computation as to how much time you have before you run out.

If you anticipate there will be only a day or so delay on the back order, you can rest easy. You can keep close watch on the diminishing supply volume and if necessary call the supply house for further knowledge concerning the length of time of the delay.

If your supplies are running out, you can immediately call some other supply firm and see if they have the product. If they do, even at a slightly higher price, your doctor may wish for you to order it from them. If no one in the area seems to have it, and you are afraid of trying a mail-order house at this late data, you had better plan to find a substitute product. After all, there is very little in the way of dental supplies on the market that does not have a competitive product somewhere. If this proves unavailable or unacceptable for your doctor, borrow from another dentist, and let him worry about running out. If you do borrow some, make sure you order an extra amount from the supplier next time in order to be able to pay him back and still keep your own schedule going at a normal pace.

Shopping

One of the beautiful advantages of the local supply house, with its regular salesmen, is dependability. They are always there when you need them, and they nearly always have what you want. If they do not have it, they will usually try very hard to get it for you. However, you must be willing to pay something for this dependability, and this can affect the price you may have to pay for a specific item.

Another advantage of the local supplyman is that he frequently will deliver free of charge any supplies you have ordered, especially the large bulk orders. There is also simplification in ordering everything from one man who calls regularly on your office every week or so.

However, your doctor may well feel that he is quite content to forego the simplicity, free delivery, and dependability in order to get a monetary gain. This is his decision alone. Your job is to aid him in his decisions and to provide him with all possible sources of information. The way to best do this is to shop through the multitude of mail-order dental catalogues that come into your office each year. You can spot a "special" and quick-check its price against your usual figure and then if it looks good, look further. If postage is to be added to the mail-order house's price, you will need to know how much weight it will have, and how much postage you may have to pay. Some houses will pay your postage for you, but not all, so be sure before you buy. If you are still of the opinion that this a a good buy, make sure you will not have to purchase so much of a particular product that its shelf-life will run out before you get a chance to use it all up.

You most certainly will want to be able to assure the doctor that the quality of the product is as good as what he is now using. If it might not possibly be as good, you can always (with doctor's permission) write the mail-order supplier for a sample to examine. If necessary, and the purchase price seems quite good in all aspects, you might want to order, say, one tube at what may be an even higher price than you are already paying, in order to try it out.

Do not overlook the mailing and delivery time expected from the supplier. Remember, mail strikes can affect your delivery.

If you have found a product from an outside house, and are quite happy with it and the price, it will never hurt to ask your local regular dental supply company if they will meet the same price. They can only say yes or no. It might be they can meet it if you will buy a larger number or quantity than usual. If this is so, but you do not have room for it in your office, ask them if they will allow you to buy it at this special price, but deliver to you only a specified certain amount at any one time.

It may well pay you to inquire into the price of some of your more commonly used items at houses outside your local area—regular established supply houses that do not cover you in their territory. It may be they would enjoy having you as an occasional buyer.

Whenever shopping, always expressly spell out exactly what you want to buy, and how much, and the size container, and the expected delay for delivery, and every specific you can think of. In this way you will avoid getting something substituted that you do not actually want. You can always send it back, but that just involves extra time, as well as additional postage expense.

6

A Dependable System for Monthly Billings and Collections

Which Type System Is Best for You?

One of the most worrisome chores in the dental office is that of making up and mailing the monthly statements. This can require anywhere from one-half to two or three days of your time, and will leave little time for anything else. In other words, all other activities of the business office must stop while the bills are being prepared. Another possibility is that you develop a severe headache trying to make out the statements, answer the telephone, go back to the statements, pull a chart for the doctor, back to the bills, schedule a patient, back to the chore—and then you knock over the pile and lose your place. Talk about stress situations! Well, let us look into doing something to make your time an easier one.

First, how do you handle your billing? A neat way is the individually typed bill, but it is unfortunately also the most time-consuming. If your dentist prefers that you continue with this type of statement, then perhaps he will at least let you use the kind that is printed in rolls. You can order these from various commercial printing houses serving the professions. You start a roll into your typewriter; type one, and tear it off along a perforated line, and then move to your next one. This will certainly speed things up, but it does unfortunately leave the rather ragged perforated edge to the statement which is not too neat. It will help if you also have windowed envelopes arranged so all you need to do is type one, tear it off and insert it into the envelope. There will be no need to type the patient's name on the envelope this way.

If you are only a fair typist, you may wish to handwrite all of your statements, and speed things up this way. However, if you do, make sure your handwriting is particularly neat and legible. You should also check with your doctor to make certain he does not object to your treating the statements this way.

Now you have to place stamps on the envelopes. This in itself can be a time-consuming task so perhaps we can speed it up for you. Try one of the following ideas:

First, you can purchase envelopes at the post office that are prestamped, and then have your doctor's name and address printed on them. A problem here is that the envelopes available are not of the finest quality and look pretty cheap. It is also impossible to obtain windowed envelopes from the post office. So you gain time in stamping, but lose time in preparing the bills.

You may wish to buy your stamps in rolls instead of sheets. In this way you can lick and stamp the envelopes more easily and quicker. Perhaps you would like to call your local office supply store and purchase a special hand machine that carries a roll of stamps and enables you to roll them out one at a time and stamp your envelopes this way. It is assumed that you use a moistened sponge rather than your tongue. You do, don't you?

Another added chore is the sealing of the bill envelopes. A moistened sponge is very easy to set up and quite cheap, but you may well find it to your advantage to purchase a special sealer at your local stationery store or office supply house. This handy apparatus will moisten the envelopes much more evenly and smoothly than you can possibly do by hand and thus speed things up as well as help you keep the entire stack neater.

The most advanced setup is to have a Pitney-Bowes postage meter machine to use. This will run into some slight expense for your doctor, to be sure, but will reduce your sealing and stamping time to an absolute minimum. It will moisten the envelope, then stamp it, then seal it—all automatically. It is most economical to get one with a hand crank, and it is still very convenient, although there are electrically driven ones available, at added expense. The electrically driven machines are handy in the sense that you do not need to do anything except feed the envelope (with the bill already inside) into the machine, but frankly, your right hand is not busy anyway, and since it is cheaper and almost as fast, you are usually better off with the hand-operated meter machine.

The way it is handled is this: your doctor either buys or leases (with some variations) the basic machine. This part has all the gears, water reservoir, and such stuff. Then there is the meter section that carries the postage. Actually, it does not hold stamps as such, but simply is a type of adding (or rather, subtracting) machine that prints figures. It must be taken to the local post office to be "filled." There they will accept your money and set up the machine to "hold" that much postage. Now you have purchased your postal stamps.

This part of the machine is reinstalled in the meter machine, and you set up, say, eight cents for each letter you wish to mail, Now, with every turn of the crank, each envelope is sealed and stamped with the preset amount of postage. The meter subtracts each eight cents (or whatever amount you have set) until the original amount of postage is used up. Then you again must return the meter to the post office with more money for the purchase of more postage.

It is usually advantageous to buy postage in at least one hundred dollar amounts, and thereby reduce the number of trips you must make to the post office. It usually takes the post office official about twenty minutes to insert the postage into your machine.

If you have a Thermofax or 3-M type billing machine available, your making up of the bills will be a breeze. An entire month's billing can then be done in practically no time at all. You simply keep a running statement of each family's account during the entire month on a special financial record card, and by using the various machines available, in essence, take a picture of the record card. This copy you send to the patient.

You can run one every four seconds. The patient gets an exact copy of your record, and this might save you some telephone explanations about his bill. (On the other hand, your doctor may not wish to send out itemized statements, so you would not do well with this system in such case.)

How about the so-called "pegboard system"? This method utilizes multiple carbons or NCR paper, and attempts to reduce writing duplication to a minimum. In the process you also record the daily charges on the patient's ledger card at the same time you are noting it on your day sheet. Thus, at the end of the month you have already recorded the accumulated fees made to that patient, and his bill is already prepared. It is a very simple procedure, then, to insert this into your envelope and mail. It is a fine system for most dental offices. Many offices simply hand the bill to the patient at his last visit to the office that particular month.

The advent of the computer billing system has brought about the removal of billing from the dental office. That is, for normal billing. You simply send a copy of your day sheet to the computing headquarters and all billing is done automatically. No fuss, no bother. The patient can receive a complete, itemized bill, or a simple, nonitemized one. It is certainly the easiest system of all for you as the dental secretary.

However, it can well be the most expensive for your doctor. There is usually a basic "installation fee" and then a set monthly fee and a set charge per statement. The big question comes as to whether or not it is cheaper to have you, the secretary, do the bills, or to have the computer do them. Each office must decide for itself.

One fine advantage of the computer is that in addition to the billing, your doctor can also receive a complete analytical breakdown and summary of the business production, collections, overhead, and in addition, the recall system can be included. It is an advantage if your doctor has the time or the desire to utilize all of the wealth of information furnished him, but it can certainly be a waste if it goes unused.

A number of commercial firms offer this type of service, as well as many of the larger banks around the country.

How to Remove the End-of-the-Month Pressure

If you have decided on the best system (or rather, if your doctor has decided), then you will usually still have that pressure of making up, enveloping, stamping, sealing and mailing. It can still become rather overwhelming even if you have everything absolutely streamlined.

This pressure can be reduced considerably if you want to do so by utilizing a technique made common by the credit card companies. That is cyclical billing, or rotation billing. Here you mail the bills of, for example, all the A's through I's, on the tenth of the month; J's through R's, on the twentieth; and S's through Z's on the thirtieth. This way you will spread out the chore and create a little less havoc between the twenty-fifth and the thirtieth. Or, you could begin on, say, the fifth of each month, and send out the A's, the B's on the sixth, C's on the seventh, and so forth. Your weekends are a hindrance here, but since there are relatively so few, it should not really be much of a bother. It would not usually be a good idea to begin your alphabet on the first of the month, due to a usual rush of more checks coming in about this time, and you might need extra time to keep up with your posting.

Another method is to follow the system used by pegboards, as discussed in the first section of this chapter. Make up the patient's bill as you go along, adding each daily fee as it accumulates, and then you will have less trouble at the end of the month.

This can become rather burdensome and a real problem if you do not actually use a pegboard, so be careful not to let a single day go by without recording a patient's fee to his bill. Remember too that there are days when you are hard pressed to finish all your regular chores, or even days when you are not present at work at all. This system requires diligent watching and care to avoid slip-ups, but can, if operated properly, reduce a great deal of your end-of-month pressure.

The Word Is Accuracy

It really seems a little ridiculous to mention accuracy to the professional dental secretary, but let's face it, people do make mistakes! After working at the same busy job day after day, it is bound to get a little boring, and errors can creep in more easily when you are bored. In addition, you are certainly familiar with the busy, busy day when about twice as many patients as normal must be seen, and you have more duties than normal. This is when you will be more susceptible to making errors than usual. This is when you accidentally record the check you received on the wrong "Smith's" chart. Or when you fail to record it at all. Or maybe it's when you write down $48 instead of the proper $84.

The most important advice that can be given to you is to take note of your busy, busy day and remember that your errors are more likely then. Now you will be able to think out slightly more clearly each item you record. You will realize that every single recording you make may be wrong, and you will naturally be more on your guard against this.

It may help you if you can sort of look twice at each recording you make, and notice whether or not it seems in perspective. For instance, does the doctor *normally* charge, say, $48 for a crown? Or does he *usually* charge $84 for an examination? Or, why would Mr. Jones pay $84 when his bill was only $48? Or, perhaps, why would he pay only $48 on a bill of $84? Most people (excluding previously arranged accounts) would pay, say, half or a third, or some relatively evenly divided sum—in this case, $42 (one-half of $84). So, continually watch for these little red flag warnings of something that doesn't quite fit. If you will think about this day after day, you will soon get into the feel of things, and then it will be easier for you to sense an error.

The Debtor List: Its Importance

As you are well aware, in every dental office there are certain patients who either do not pay or else pay very slowly.

There are usually only a few of these people, but they will create most of your collection headaches. We must see if we can reduce some of the problems.

Do this: start and keep a regular debtor list. When you get a chance to do so, go down your ledger cards, and make an alphabetical list of all patients who owe you money. Record the name, the amount and the date of their last payment. This will obviously take some time if you have a hundred or more patients, so plan your time when you can spare it. If you keep it up regularly, you will only need to make up this list once.

A running summary such as in Figure 6-1 will quickly help you to spot the slow payers. Their names will continually keep coming back up on the list, month after month. This summary will also give you a quick total outstanding check.

What you have here then is a list of all those patients that owe you (the dentist, actually) money. As each patient pays his bill, you can cross out his name. You also add new names as they occur during the month. When you send out the bills at the end of the month (or whenever), you can double check if you wish, and make sure that your list is still accurate.

Around the tenth of the following month you pull out your list and look to see whose names are still on the list. These people are beginning to be slow payers. About the fifteenth you will have more evidence, and if by the twentieth there are still some patients who have bills that remain unpaid from the previous month, then you are to pay particular attention to them the upcoming month.

Now you run your end-of-the-month double check with your billing again. Anyone whose name is still on the original list is now definitely over thirty days behind. Your job at this point is to notify your doctor that these certain patients are overdue on their accounts. Let him decide if he wishes for you to take any action now.

You should continue this add-and-cross-off list from month to month. Remember to take note of the month that you add

DEBTOR LIST

Name	Phone	Amount	Last Paid
Abbott, J. W.	123-4567	$ 24	12/12/71
Adams, R. L.	234-5678	10	8/ 4/71
Beaver, H. H.	345-6789	125	10/ 5/71
Deacol, M. X.	456-7890	14	8/13/71
Everettes, K. L.	567-8912	365	12/10/71
Mills, Miss Billie	678-9012	6	1/ 3/72
Oxfort, Niles	789-0123	46	6/28/71
Rapporflosia, Bill	890-1234	531	1/27/72
Whositte, S. O.	901-2345	5	7/21/71

Figure 6-1

each name. Soon you will note that there are certain names that remain on the list from month to month. Action must be taken on these patients.

The Best Way to Handle the Budget Agreement

One of your more pleasant collection chores is that of overseeing the budget accounts. That is, it is pleasant if you have done your job correctly from the beginning. If you have, then ninety-nine percent of your budget accounts will come in every month and on schedule. You can count on them.

The key is to start them off right in the beginning. You must gently but firmly take each patient by the hand (figuratively) and guide him through to the correct decisions for setting up his budget plan.

The mistake most offices make is to set it up so that the patient is in financial strain. That is to say, either the initial payment is set so high that the patient may have to borrow elsewhere in order to meet it, and then have to pay that back monthly, while trying to make regular monthly payments to you, too.

At other times the patient is set up with monthly payments so high that he cannot make them with any regularity. He will usually make the first one, or maybe two, but all the while he is putting off someone else. Then they get on his back and he pays them instead of you. And your doctor's budget gets out of whack because some money he was counting on did not come in.

Now some doctors are certainly more adamant about the strictness of the budget plans in their office than others, and they have a right to run their office any way they see fit. If, however, your doctor will permit a more liberal monthly (or weekly) budget plan, then here is what you will want to do:

First, you obtain the total projected cost to the patient—the fee. You should try to obtain this from the doctor at the first appointment if at all possible. It is best if you can establish good paying habits with the patient while he is having his work done. He has dentistry and its benefits on his mind and will have much more incentive to pay then than later when he has not even been in the office for some time.

Now sit down with the patient and spell out in general terms the basics of your own office's budget plan. Say something to the effect that, "There is the required initial payment" or "retainer" or even "down payment." Actually "down payment" usually has such a commercial and nonprofessional tone to it, that it is generally felt that it is not in good taste to say it here. So you say that after the initial payment, the balance may be paid over several months. At this point you should emphasize that there is "no additional cost or finance charge" (assuming that there are actually none).

You should say that while there is no specific requirement in this very flexible budget program, most patients with cases of this size will make an initial payment of about —————. And here you mentally calculate in round numbers one-third or one-fourth (or whatever your doctor really prefers) of the total fee. The best down payment amount from your office's standpoint is one that will at least pay the anticipated laboratory bills for this particular patient. Most dentists determine a fee by tripling or quadrupling the laboratory bill. Therefore a third or a fourth of the total will usually just about pay the laboratory. Try to get this amount when feasible.

I'd say to the patient, "Do you feel that you can comfortably make an initial payment of somewhere in this neighborhood?" If the patient says yes, then you can proceed, but if he says he cannot, you should ask, "What amount do you feel you can pay?" If you can interject into the conversation enough influence and friendly guidance to keep the initial payment as high as possible, then fine, but if this patient simply does not have it, accept what he can pay.

By the way, you have already checked out his credit references, haven't you? And found no reasons to doubt that he should be extended credit? You should be doing this while the doctor is examining the patient if today is the first visit that patient has made to this office.

Once you have set down the initial payment amount, decide when it is to be paid—preferably today, but never later than the day the doctor is to begin the major work. If the patient says he will not be able to pay the initial payment until next month, then you had better accept this fact, but why not casually set his first appointment conveniently on that particular date? You need not make a big production out of it—it is just standard policy of the office to begin the major work the day the initial payment is made.

If the patient is having a specific area of discomfort and cannot wait, then certainly your doctor will gladly place a temporary filling or so to hold him until his first major appointment.

Always remember that these patients of ours rarely realize how much expense they will have to undergo, and very few people will have set aside sufficient funds, so you should try to be as lenient as practical and still adhere to good business principles.

Now you must determine the amount of the monthly (or weekly, or bi-weekly) payment. Whether it is weekly, bi-weekly or monthly or whatever should coincide with the timing of the patient's pay check. It is rather ridiculous to have a patient set up on a weekly pay schedule when he only gets paid monthly, isn't it?

First take the total and subtract the initial payment and you are left with the balance. If you normally will spread the payments over six months, divide six into this last figure and you have the basic payment. Ask the patient if this figure is reasonable in relation to his budget. If you feel he might be able to do so, why not divide four into the balance, and strive for four months? Or even three. But you must be absolutely positive the patient will be comfortable with this amount of monthly payment, because if he is not, you just might not get it all or at least on the schedule you propose.

If Mr. Jones says he cannot make even six months, try asking what he had in mind, and perhaps the two of you can get together on a better figure this way. You may need, in some instances, to extend the payments over to eight or even ten months in order to make arrangements. If your doctor will accept this then fine, because you will be enabling the patient to obtain good dentistry when he needs it, not necessarily when he can afford it. Just make sure you do not overextend any patient more than necessary, and be certain not to spread out so many cases that you doctor cannot afford to continue.

A good rule to follow is: the more the initial payment, the smaller the monthly payment can be and the longer the monthly payments can be spread out. Conversely, the smaller the initial payment, the larger the monthly payments should be. Remember, though, that each patient may require specifically different payment arrangements just as he may require different types of dentistry.

Many patients are paying monthly for various home appliances and may wish to carry smaller monthly payments with you until they finish paying on something else. In this case, you should always have at least a token payment from them each month—and place it all in writing—until they can increase the budget payments with your office.

Always give your patient some choice as to the date the payments are due at your office. You may certainly suggest a couple of dates, say the third or the eighteenth for the convenience of the office. Ask him if either of these dates is satisfactory. If not, then you should let the patient tell you his most satisfactory date for payment. After all, if the patient cannot conveniently meet his obligation to your office on time, then you are just asking for headaches in collections.

The Importance of the Follow-Up

One of the real keys to eliminating collection problems is the follow-up. This means simply that if you have a prearranged date on which a certain patient is scheduled to pay his budget account and you do not receive his money on that day, you must follow it up immediately. You must call or write him *the day after* his payment failed to arrive.

An important note here is that right away the patient comes to the realization that he is dealing with an office that, while reasonable and liberal with its budget plan, is still absolutely and strictly professional and businesslike. He knows he must pay on time as originally scheduled. He now knows that he is expected to uphold his end of the contract to the letter.

But what if you call and he says he mailed it yesterday? Well that's fine. He now has to realize that he will have to mail it a day earlier, since you have pointed out to him that his payment did not arrive on schedule and is now a date late. You, of course, will always be quite pleasant when calling such patients.

If you continue to call each and every patient—*every* time a payment does not arrive on time, pretty soon word will get around that the payment plan in your office is strictly business and no sloppy payment habits will be tolerated.

You should never be embarrassed to call these patients because after all, they have been given the basic decision as to when the payment is due in your office. If you need an excuse, you can always say your accountant insists that you keep accurate records and reports. If someone is late with his payment, then you must show it on your records,and then you catch it from both the doctor and his accountant.

If a patient consistently sends his payments late, and you constantly must call, you might try writing a formal letter. In this letter you can suggest better adherence to the terms of "item three" (or whatever) of his budget plan contract—where he said he would make payments on or before such and such a date each month.

If you still get no further results this way, and his payments continue to come in late, then you should call the patient directly and ask him if he prefers to change his payment date to a more convenient one. It may be that his personal finances have changed, and he would welcome a chance to get his account straightened out. And it will eliminate your headache—at least this one!

The Need for Tact

When dealing with people concerning their payments—particularly late or missed payments, you frequently run into someone with a very nasty attitude about the whole thing, such as trying to put you on the defensive for having the audacity to call or getting so nasty as to hang up in your ear, or even cursing you. It takes a special kind of dental secretary to handle people like this. Let's try to make you that special gal!

The key words are tact and patience. With both of these on your side, you are bound to be able to best just about anyone in a difficult conversation. It is not easy to know which of the two is more important, so you might say you need fifty-one percent tact and fifty-one percent patience.

You must always remember that in your job as collection agent you must always keep things in perspective. You must never, never lose your temper. Realize that things people may say to you from time to time are so rude and insulting as to put your self-control to its utmost test, but remember, it takes two to make an argument, and know this well: an argument between a patient and a dental auxiliary is strictly a no-no.

Keep it well in mind that in reality you are the doctor's extra hand and voice. The tasks and details that you do for him are his own choosing. He could just as well be speaking to this patient instead of you. You can be quite sure your dentist would not want to jeopardize his chances for collecting a bill with a simple loss of temper. (On the other hand, perhaps he doesn't mind winning an argument and losing some dollars, but certainly not as a general rule!)

The point here is that to keep your chances of collecting a slow or bad bill alive, you must keep the patient's thoughts about the office and staff as pleasant as you can make them under the circumstances. Very few patients are true dead beats and actually try to get dentistry done with no prior intention to pay the bill. Basic human nature tells us that we would rather be able to meet our financial obligations and have the respect of others. It is just that sometimes people cannot quite meet all their expenses and must have some extra consideration. After all, how many of us can accurately anticipate medical and/or dental expenses?

Most patients will pay their accounts—even if only very slowly—if you can present to them an understanding attitude. You can tactfully suggest that they offer as little as one dollar a week as a token payment on just about any size bill. This will at least give them an opportunity to show you and the dentist their good faith about honoring their legitimate debt. Here is where patience enters the picture on the part of your doctor. He must be willing to accept such a tiny token payment from this patient.

You must tactfully let the patients realize that you are sympathetic with their financial pressures, but keep them well aware of their dental bill with you. If you insult them or offend them, you are more likely to be shut off completely. All some people need is just the slightest excuse not to pay and "that's all folks." The patient says to himself, "She treated me like dirt, so I'll not pay them at all!" Beware of the tone of your voice at all times. Just a slight sneering inflection can sound very cruel to a patient who is already embarrassed and upset over being called about his account.

You're probably familiar with the guy who does not pay and when you call him, he complains that something was wrong with the dentistry he had done by your doctor. Oh sure, he's had it for nine months and has never called to let you know he was dissatisfied, but now you know. Boy, does he ever let you have it about your doctor's lousy work!

Just listen patiently, and listen, and listen to all he has to say. Be sure to jot down the highlights of his complaints so you can relay this to the dentist. Now after Mr. Grouch has run his course, pleasantly inform him that the doctor stands behind all of his work. Point out that had the doctor known Mr. Grouch was dissatisfied, he would have done something about it immediately. You will want to follow with an appointment at the earliest possible moment the patient will come in. Remember, it might just be that he does have a legitimate gripe, and your employer will most graciously correct the situation. *Note:* The dissatisfied patient spreads word of his dissatisfaction almost more than the happy patient spreads his good word.

If Mr. Grouch does not want to come in to have it corrected, but wants you to drop the bill, you need to lay it in your doctor's lap. It will become his decision whether or not he wishes to pursue the matter. It sometimes can become a touchy legal situation, and many lawsuits have become instigated this way. Just be careful to say nothing to the patient that would offend him any more. Be pleasant even if it hurts you inside. Never give any patient any excuse to criticize your office.

If you have to call some patient and she goes into such a tirade as to make a complete fool of herself, do not "twist the dagger." Do not push the issue of her foolishness. Just ignore it, say pleasantly and courteously what you need to say, and finish the conversation. There is no need for comments to her about her attitude or opinions. All you want to do is to get the bill paid in as easy and pleasant a way as possible.

When to Give Up

The point at which you finally turn the patient over to a collection agency is never a clear-cut one. There are certain basics to follow, but you must always bear in mind that you are dealing with people and that every one is a slightly different situation.

Let us assume that you have run your gauntlet. You have called this patient several times to no avail. You have run through all of your standard collection letters and still you have had no results. The patient has said he would pay it, and yet would give you no time as to when, and will not make any type of small token payment. What next?

Make one last telephone call (or letter if he has moved away) and pleasantly but firmly tell him that if he cannot make some effort of good will to show that he does actually intend to pay the bill, that you will have to suggest to your dentist that the account be placed with a collection agency. You need to remind the patient that one bad credit report can prevent him from borrowing money from a bank or home loan mortgage association. A bad credit report can, in fact, ruin a man's life.

If you still hear nothing from your patient after this, you should definitely follow through and contact your local collection agency about him. Always be certain, however, to let the doctor make the final decision about this.

7 | *Controlling Accounts, Accountant, and Accounting*

The Requirements

Bookkeeping is a vital part of every dental office whether you like it or not. Believe me, most of us would rather not mess with paperwork. This is one of the main reasons dentists hire dental assistants to do the dull jobs for them! Keeping the office books can be dull as creation or you can make it rather exciting—your preference entirely.

Now why do we have bookkeeping anyway? The foremost answer is money, and the second reason is to stay friendly with Uncle Sam. We must always know how much money people owe us so we can collect the proper amounts. In addition, the Internal Revenue Service likes to have you prove how much money your office made every once in a while, so you need lots of records for this.

You must keep total and complete recordings of every monetary transaction made in the office. This is really needed to help your doctor run his business. He needs to know if he has a going concern. He needs to know if he should increase his working time or his fees, or if he needs to emphasize payments more to his patients. In other words, without proper bookkeeping it is difficult or impossible to stay in business.

The Internal Revenue Service looks with suspicion on anyone with poor or incomplete records. Their opinion: anyone with professional training and intelligence who keeps poor books is easily susceptible to error and to not reporting his total income for taxation. So two words must become your guide: thoroughness and accuracy.

Your doctor depends on you to maintain every financial recording of his business. He has provided you with ample record forms for this purpose, so make sure you follow through accordingly. He, likewise, has provided you with an adding machine or the equivalent, so there can be no excuse for errors save carelessness. Incidentally, the IRS doesn't excuse carelessness, so it is highly unlikely your employer will either. If he has an error on his income tax that is not in the government's favor, he is penalized and charged interest. You'd better hope your boss will not decide to charge you for your errors! Plus interest.

Which Forms, How and When?

Generally speaking, there are too many different individual forms to go into here for general bookkeeping. Each dental office will have its preferred ones and you can easily adapt to each one. Some will have daily work sheets with a column for production and another for collections. Other dentists ignore the productions column completely and concentrate on the collection side, considering collection to be the amount of work done. Either way is fine as long as you are accurate with all computations and recordings.

The Monthly Depository

If your dentist pays at least $200 each quarter in withholding tax and social security taxes, he is required to make a monthly deposit to either the IRS or a local "Federal Depository" bank. In this way the revenue people feel there is less chance of an employee getting excessively far behind on his payments of the amount withheld, and social security taxes and the employees can be better assured of having been properly taken care of. If their taxes are not paid by their employer, they might not receive all of their anticipated benefits later.

So, once a month, you must make out a Form 501 and sent it along with a check from your doctor's office account for the payment. It is due on the fifteenth of each month for February, March, May, June, August, September, November, and December and on the last day of the month in January, April, July, and October. On these latter four months, a Form 941 is required.

To figure out the amount due with Form 501, take the total withheld from each employee's salary for the preceding month, for example, $50. Now take the amount withheld for FICA (social security tax), say, $20. The employer has to pay this same amount out of his pocket, so add $20, then add this total of $40 to the withheld $50, and you arrive at $90, which is the amount to be deposited along with the filled out Form 501. Make sure you always send the entire card along with the check, so you can get the receipt stub back for your records.

How to Compute the Quarterly Return

Each quarter the final check is deposited as usual at the bank or it can be mailed into your regional center with the completed Form 941. On this form are the names, social security numbers and salaries of all employees, and the general tabulation of the quarter's deposits.

Make sure you make these deposits on schedule since there is that usual penalty (monetary) if you are late. If the fifteenth or the last day of the month or quarter comes on a Saturday or Sunday or on a national holiday, you can wait until the following day, but really, why push it?

The Doctor's Quarterly Estimate

Your doctor pays income taxes just the same as everyone else. More than likely, though, he must make payments every quarter. This means that every three months he must compute (or have his accountant or dental assistant do it for him) the amount of federal income tax he expects to have to pay for the year in progress, and then pay roughly one-fourth of it. Here again, Uncle Sam is concerned that the average guy just might not be able to accumulate the total during the year and pay it totally on time. In addition, the government likes to have some money coming in regularly during the year. Anyway, once each quarter the doctor must run a projected estimate on how much he will net during the year and how much tax he should have to pay. Your part of this is to have (and keep readily available) an up-to-date figure of collections thus far this year (total) and a summarized total of office expenditures. Therefore, the doctor can take the collections thus far, subtract the expenditures, and have a net profit figure. It is this figure that you should provide for him each month if he wishes it. It is his profit (or loss). He then will multiply this by four, if it is in April, double it if in June, or add one-fourth of it in September in order to project ahead to the end of the year. Then he will substract his personal deductions and exemptions and arrive at the final estimated figure upon which his tax base and percentage are established. He will want to review it closely each quarter, because frequently the rate of net profit will change during the year and he must (by law) estimate within seventy percent of accuracy. If he is under on his estimate, he will be penalized.

The final estimate is made on January 15, so his last chance to bring the total estimate up to within seventy percent is then. His final tax is paid on April 15, just like yours, and only minor adjustments up or down are usually made then, because he must also pay the first payment of the new year's estimate then.

Some states require rather stringent adherence to similar rules, so be sure you check with your doctor or his accountant about local and state rules.

The Annual Tax—How It Concerns You

Prior to April 15, your doctor will be having his final state and federal income tax figured. This is usually done over several weeks prior to his basic meeting with his accountant. He will be gathering, and searching, and searching again for any type of legal deductions he can find. This is where the top-notch dental secretary can help tremendously.

You must start by knowing that any legitimate expense in running the business is tax deductible. This covers the salaries, utilities, supplies, and such, but you must keep diligent track of each tiny expenditure made even down to the penny you gave the postman for postage due; each tip you gave a delivery boy; that time you gave little Johnny bus fare home from his dental appointment. And don't forget that day you bought the 10¢ box of labels for the doctor at the local five and dime. You must have a written record of every penny you spend for the doctor in every manner. The dentist must be able to show in black and white proof of each and every expenditure he makes, just as he must also be able to show proof of his collections.

If you faithfully will keep a book of all tiny, cash expenditures during the year, your doctor will be able to take one look at it, total it and have all the information in an instant. This is far better than having to search the entire office over in fear of missing something, isn't it?

A point to remember here is that if your doctor makes a check out to petty cash for these expenditures, you can count them only once. You must still keep the detailed record, but he cannot deduct both the check amount and this total—only one or the other.

Always keep together invoices of supplies purchased during the year. The boss just might get audited some day and he will have to prove to the IRS agents that he did actually purchase everything he claims he did. Keep a special file folder marked "Paid Bills," and place everything here. Keep the years separate, however; never let one year's invoices get stuck into another's. You'd never find them again. At the end of each year, pack up all of the paid bills and label them carefully and stash them away somewhere. Be sure to tell your doctor where you have placed them.

A convenient storage bin is one of these "bill boxes" from the local stationery store that have the outside appearance of a large book. They come in uniform sizes and will usually hold a year's supply and will store easily. Label the outside in detail. If you have too much material for one "book," separate the dental supplies from the rest. They are usually the major purchases made during the year. You could itemize these supply invoices by company if you wish.

If you do have more than one box or package to pack up, be certain that when you label them you note clearly on the back—"Box 1 of 2"; or "Box 2 of 2." In this manner you or anyone else will know to look for another box or package somewhere. (They should ideally be tied together.)

The Checkbook Reconciliation

One of the most frustrating moments a person can have is when you find that your checkbook balance does not agree with that of the bank. We've all had this happen from time to time and it can be hair-raising. Simply speaking, it is only necessary to step-by-step discover a missed check, deposit or math error. But often you can become bogged down in a myriad of numbers and lose yourself completely.

Since it is part of your job to keep the doctor's papers in order and frequently you have charge of the checkbook, you must know how to reconcile it quickly and smoothly.

First: get all the checks and place them in numerical order. Now flip them down one by one and record each one that is absent. Remember that you will usually have a few that were missing from the previous month to check off first. I suggest that you place a small red check beside the check number on each check stub in the checkbook as you flip through the checks.

When you have recorded the numbers of all missing checks, jot down the amounts of these checks and then total them. This is the amount that has not yet cleared the bank.

Now check your notation of all deposits made during the month with those shown on the bank statement. You should have a duplicate slip or ticket for each day's deposit. Many banks will return your originals to you, but others do not, so keep all of your duplicates. If you have made any deposits that have not yet shown up on the bank's records, note this.

Begin with the final balance as recorded by the bank and note the amount. Add any deposits that you have made that do not appear on the statement. Total. Next subtract the total from above of the checks that have not yet cleared the bank. Total.

Now look over the statement and find any service charges made and subtracted from your doctor's account. Some banks charge nothing if you keep a certain minimum balance each month, but always check anyway; even banks make errors occasionally. If there is a service charge, go back to your checkbook and subtract it from the account balance after the last check.

At this point your checkbook balance should equal the bank statement balance.

They don't? Okay, here's what to do. First, double check everything you have done. Do it all again. Did you skip a check? A deposit? Did you add the service charge instead of subtracting? Did you subtract it again from the bank statement balance?

Still can't find the error? Next start back in your checkbook at the beginning figure for the month, and double check all math. Run a tape on every deposit and check, subtract the service charge and see if you balance this time. Were there any bank drafts you overlooked? Did the bank make any debit memos (say for new checks) you failed to see?

Okay, next look at each check and compare its figure with that of the check stub. Are they the same? Did you write 1.01 on one and 1.04 on the other?

Is it possible the bank mistook your numerals for others? You'll need to cross-check the figures on each check (you've already checked out the stubs) against the figures recorded for the checks on the bank statement. Sometimes 0's look like 6's and vice versa, and 4's look like 7's or 9's or even 1's, or occasionally 2's. Double check the bank statement math.

Once you finally arrive at the corrected reconciliation, place a double line under the correct balance in the checkbook and label it "correct," and the date, and your initials. *Never* do this if you are not absolutely positive you do have it correct. An error here could throw off the balancing for months.

The Posting Technique

Just a brief note on posting because this can vary so widely with each office. The word—as always—is accuracy. You must never permit yourself to get so rushed at posting time that you get careless and/or sloppy. You should always take ample time to think of what you are doing as you are doing it. That is, do not intend to write $4.00 and write $40.00; or do not intend to write 4 and have it come out looking like 7.

Likewise try hard not to pull James Brom's chart when you really wanted James Brown's, or Jim Brown's. Are you certain you have the correct William Jamerson? There may be two, remember.

Just as you had May Smith's chart out and were ready to post, the telephone rang. Then you put her chart away unposted. That is a no-no, isn't it?

Again, take time to think as you work. Do not let it all become so automatic that you get so you cannot remember what you did or did not do.

A good tip is to place a small check beside the patient's name on the daily record sheet as soon as you have completed the posting to the chart. This way the absence of a check would be a key to go back to the chart and double check.

How to Help the Doctor's Accountant

In order to serve the dentist best, you need to do everything in your capability to make things run smoothly around the entire office. This applies also to his accountant. Whether the accountant comes into the office or all of the pertinent information is sent out to him, you can be a real key to victory over a difficult chore.

Be neat and a stickler for details, that's the secret. The accountant will be gathering hundreds of various figures from a multitude of sources, and this can frequently be a backbreaking job. Small wonder so many accountants wear glasses—after looking at small numbers all day (and many nights).

Know your office like the inside of your hand. Keep a close watch on your filing system, so that if the accountant (or even the doctor) should request a specific letter, statement, bill, or invoice, you will know exactly where to find it. This is efficiency via expert knowledge. Never be found wasting your time and especially the accountant's looking—searching—the files for an item he needs. Catalogue your files so that they are readily understandable to any stranger in the room. Make sure they are alphabetized (I mean the general, miscellaneous file—not the patients' records file), and it is a good idea to have a typed listing of just what files you do have, so your doctor will know. He shouldn't have to waste his time some night fumbling through the files hunting for something pertinent to an order or invoice.

The slip of the files should be outlined to have the major headings, but should also be broken down into some subheadings. For instance, under the major file under "correspondence" you could have (1) "employment," (2) "patient," (3) "personal," and so on.

Keep your financial records neat. If you make an error, don't mark it all through so as to be illegible. Simply mark one line through the middle, e.g., ($300.10). This way your page will be neat, and the exact type of error will be clear to the accountant.

Do not let your words or especially your figures run together. Try to keep them about the same size (not too small) so they will be easy to read.

Make sure your pencil is always sharp, or your pen clear.

If your office hires a new accountant, one of the first things you need to do is to show him some of your handwriting and make sure it is legible to him. It makes little difference how neat and accurate you are if your writing cannot be read by the accountant.

Watch out for carbon paper and/or dirty smudges. And never lose any important records!

If you can follow through with all of these suggestions and thoughts, you and the accountant should have smooth sailing.

The Case
Presentation

Your Purpose

If your doctor gives a formal (or even an informal) presentation of the patient's case, you can be of tremendous value to him. It is here that the proper attitude and word by you can totally convince the patient to approve the doctor's recommended program.

Quite frequently the patient is not really sure just what to do. Even if the spouse has been right there for the presentation, there may still be a great deal of doubt in their minds about proceeding. The doctor has just given a complete description of what he wishes to do, but the patient simply needs more reassurance and from someone other than the doctor himself. This must come from you. You are the key. What you say, and how you say it must be carefully planned and phrased in order to eliminate any lingering doubt in the patient's mind that the doctor's proposed program is best and should be accepted. You must absolutely exude confidence.

In addition, you, yourself, must have total confidence in the doctor's prescription. You must want this program as if it were for you or your husband. You know it is a fine plan or the dentist would not have proposed it. Just imagine that your mouth were in the shape of the patient's and you would wish for the finest, longest-lasting, and nicest-looking dentistry available. You would want to reduce to a minimum all possible future dental problems. You would want to get the maximum value for your health dollar. You would want the most comfortable mouth—and—the most pleasing, natural smile around anywhere.

This is what dentistry can do for you and for the patient. This is what the dentist wants to do for his patient. It is the dentist's job—whether he will admit it to himself or not—to "sell" the patient on all the tremendous advantages of fine dentistry. It therefore becomes your job and sincere duty to reinforce all of your dentist's salesmanship.

The Procedure

For the average better dental office the usual procedure goes something like this: the dentist examines the patient, uses X-rays as necessary, then either at an informal session in the chair immediately or at a formal presentation later in the private office or conference room, describes to the patient the basic problems found, and the anticipated prognosis, followed by his recommendations and alternatives, and finally quotes fee estimates for the anticipated work. At this point it is usually convenient and quite proper to dismiss himself from the patient and his spouse, so that they can discuss their decisions.

Now, after a few minutes, it is the time for you, the dental financial secretary to enter the picture. You say to Mr. and Mrs. Jones, "Doctor has been tied up with another item momentarily. Have either of you any questions concerning the dentistry that he proposed for you?"

Or, at this point, you take note of the patient's chart as to the case most strongly recommended by the doctor. He has checked the most favorable plan with his pencil as he was leaving the room, and since you had already written up the case estimates for the dentist, you should be readily familiar with each specific plan (Plan I, Plan II, Plan III, Plan IV, etc.), and a great deal of the details of each. From your own background and experience you know the advantage of each program.

If the patient has no specific questions, it is frequently a good idea to ask a specific question pertinent to the checked program, such as, "Did the doctor point out all of the advantages of a porcelain crown to you?" If Mrs. Jones says yes, you can continue to the next place by mentioning something to the effect that one of your best friends had a similar program done a few weeks (or months, etc.) ago and was *so* pleased with the results! Or you can say that you're quite sure that he will be pleased with the comfort (or chewing ability) he will receive from that fixed bridge.

Whatever you say you must never give any possible downgrading or disparaging remarks concerning the impending treatment. It is up to doctor to point out any shortcomings of the dentistry that he cares to. It is your job to reinforce the advantages. It is so very important at this stage for the patient to gain confidence in the doctor and his total office.

If the patient has any questions concerning the proposal, then you should answer each one to the best of your ability. Be honest, but remember again—it is not up to you to initiate in any way any shortcomings about the dentistry. If a patient asks you if "it will hurt," you should not say yes—ever. You might say, "There is occasionally some slight discomfort." You should also hasten to point out that doctor *always* does everything possible to minimize any discomfort on the part of the patient.

If you are asked, "What would you do?" there is only one answer you can give. It is the obvious one—"Just what the dentist recommended."

Many dental offices offer the major patients three choices. These are something like: the holding plan ("Plan I") where the decay is stopped and the teeth are filled with the minimum cost. This program "holds" the patient in status quo until something finer can be undertaken.

The optimum plan ("Plan III") offers the patient the finest that is available. When working up this program, no fees are considered. It is strictly the "Cadillac." It would contain things like precision-attached partials instead of external-clasped partials. It is the "Swissedenture" instead of the conventional denture. It is the Ceramco or Microbond crown instead of the full gold crown.

The compromise plan ("Plan II") is just what the name

TOOTH		SERVICES NECESSARY	I	II	III		
			319	920	1658		
3	1	DIST (C)	A	C	C		
	2	OCC	↓				
4	3	MES	A	A	G		
	4	OCC					
	5	DIST	↓	↓			
5	6	DIST	A	A	G		
	7	OCC	↓	↓			
7	8	DIST	S	S	S		
	9	LING	↓	↓	↓		
8	10	DIST (J)	S	J	J		
	11	LING					
	12	MES	↓				
12	13	MES	A	A	G		
	14	OCC					
	15	DIST	↓	↓			
13	16	MES (G)	A	G	G		
	17	OCC					
	18	DIST	↓				
15	19	MES	A	A	G		
	20	OCC	↓	↓			
19	21	BUC FC	FC	FC	FC		
20	22	MES	A	A	G		
	23	OCC					
	24	DIST	↓	↓			
28	25	DIST	A	A	G		
	26	OCC	↓	↓			
29	27	MES	A	A	G		
	28	OCC					
	29	DIST	↓	↓			
30	30	MES (G)	A	G	G		
	31	OCC					
	32	DIST	↓				
	33	DIAGNOSIS	DX	DX	DX		
	34	PROPHYLAXIS	PX	PX	PX		
	35						
	36						
	37						
	38						

Figure 8-1:   Case Plans

implies. It is a compromise between fine dentistry and dollars. It will treat the most seriously involved teeth properly, say, with crowns or gold inlays, and treat the less seriously affected teeth with silver amalgam.

In the example of Plans I, II and III in Figure 8-1 for a typical patient's case, note the following:

Plan I: This patient needs thirty-two separate surfaces restored. The computation also includes the original diagnosis appointment (X-rays, examination, diagnostic models, etc.) as well as a prophylaxis. Tooth #19 requires a full cast crown, whereas several others ideally should have castings, but can still accept routine amalgam or silicate restorations. The total fee is computed for all services, and comes to $319.

Plan II: This plan builds on Plan I in the sense that tooth numbers 3, 8, 13, 30 are to receive the finest treatment via castings and a porcelain jacket crown in addition to the casting on number 19. The remaining teeth receive conventional amalgams and silicates. Final computation: $920.

Plan III: This is the case treated in the finest treatment that is practicable. All teeth in the posterior are treated with castings. Number 8 will still receive a jacket. Number 7 remains silicate because a jacket is simply not indicated. Final computation: $1,658.

Mostly doctors offer all three plans to the patient, with a specific recommendation for Plan II. This starts the patient on a road to fine, long-lasting dentistry, but doesn't hit the pocketbook so hard. This is usually the plan you will find checked as you enter the conference room to speak with the patients.

Now what to say if the patient asks you, "Which plan would you choose?" You should say you would prefer the optimum plan (Plan III). After all, it is the best, isn't it? (If it is not truly the best dentistry that could be done for this patient regardless of cost, it shouldn't be listed as a possible procedure.) But if you are just absolutely positive the patient can in no way pay for Plan III, then you can point out that he should go with Plan II, for now, with the idea of working toward Plan III on a gradual basis. That is, fix the worst teeth properly now, and hold the status quo on the rest. Then in one, three or five years, whenever something additional gives way, rebuild it properly at that time. For instance, place amalgam in that molar now, and when it gives way or cracks in five years, crown it then. The patient buys some time this way. Or, rebuild that incisal angle in the central with plastic for the time being, but in three or four years, when it has discolored, or worn down, go ahead at that time with the porcelain jacket.

The point is: get the patient thinking ahead. Plant seeds of information that will develop over the years. Let him know that he will need a crown or an inlay or a jacket in a few years, and he can be better prepared for it when the time comes.

How to Get the Patient to Accept
a Better Recommendation

One of the best ways to please your employer is to have him discover that after having left you and the patient together to settle the financial arrangements, he returns to find the patient has chosen to go with a better program than the one he had suggested. This would be like leaving the room with the patient choosing to proceed with Plan I, but after discussing it with the DA, chooses Plan II, or likewise switches from Plan II to Plan III. Or perhaps just upgrading Plan I or II to something closer to the ideal.

This ability to influence the patient is one of the major keys to the successful dental team. As long as diagnoses and performances are correct, better dentistry will always be in the best health interests of the patient. Therefore, the more you can persuade a patient to accept the finest dentistry, the more he will benefit. The main difficulty is in the lack of dental education of the patient—knowledge of the real advantage of fine dentistry; and competition from the commercial industries for his dollar. It is a rare bird indeed who will willingly and happily forego that stereo, or color TV for a fixed bridge he's been needing for ten years.

The communications media today throw out the pitch for the finer life—the status—today so forcefully that we in the dental profession are frequently hard pressed to make even the slightest breakthrough with dental knowledge. Most patients dislike dentistry in the first place, and just don't care about hearing about it. They have existed with patchwork dentistry for years, and have lived with the knowledge that their parents probably wound up with dentures, and that they would too, and that's the way it is. So why bother?

Dentistry is just now beginning to make some headway against such ideas, and you DAs are the real key. Your availability to the patient for casual discussions far exceeds that of your dentist, so the major burden must fall on you, and you must accept the challenge graciously.

So for this reason, you must *always* be excited when discussing dentistry with your patients. Your cheerfulness about it, your sheer exuberance will help to break through the possible displeasure of most patients and help them to willingly make the proper decision toward fine dentistry.

Here's what you should do. When you are at your postpresentation discussion with the patient, after the dentist has complete his outline, you should briefly go over the highlights. It should go something like this: "Well, now let's see, Mr. Jones, you have chosen to have the doctor place a full gold crown on your lower molar and a fixed bridge and silver fillings for the remaining teeth. I note you have chosen to have jackets placed in your front teeth. This program comes to $535 and also includes the cleaning you will have as well as a customized program of home care. You have decided to go with a good plan and it should serve you nicely. Dr. Blank has you started on a fine plan. [This reinforces your patient's opinion of the dentist and the patient's decision to start.] I notice though, that you decided to put silver in the upper molar. It is certainly a large one. You know, you're already going with $535, and for only $80 *more* you could have the doctor go ahead with a strong, long-lasting gold inlay. I'm sure that the doctor feels that silver will serve for now or he would not have suggested it, but it would be so much nicer and after all, would only run $80 more than you're already paying."

Now here's what you have done: you have emphasized to the patient that the plan he has chosen is a good one. You have reinforced your doctor. You have also added to the patient's education. You have pointed out to the patient that for only a small amount more he can increase the total health of his mouth considerably.

Granted, you will not persuade a patient to increase his plan very often, but on the other hand, if you don't try you'll never enlarge any program. The percentages are totally in your favor.

Keep this in mind, however, that you must be somewhat

judicious in how you approach this enlargement program. Some patients may be totally offended by your approach—it may smack of "hard sell"—if you come on too strong. So always chat a moment or two with the patient to grasp his attitude about his work and its cost. If you feel he is quite contented and has readily accepted the fee, you could proceed. Hold back, though, with the patient who already seems sullen and is either there with a chip on his shoulder or a scowl on his face when you walk in.

Now if you do confront a patient who seems sullen and depressed when you begin, but who opens up when you have shown him how easily his bill can be worked out (monthly, etc.) you could easily project that for only, say $14 more per month he could go ahead and put a fine gold inlay on that upper molar ($80 divided by 6 months = $14 per month).

How to Plant Seeds

If you feel you cannot add to the patient's program in any of the aforementioned ways, try this: remind the patient that he is having the doctor place silver in that large molar in his upper right. It will certainly suffice for now, but it would no doubt be to the patient's advantage to upgrade it to a gold inlay as soon as feasible. "Therefore why not plan on having the doctor proceed with a nice gold inlay in about six or seven months, or a year. This way you can just continue making your monthly payments after your budget plan is finished and the doctor can upgrade that tooth and give it better protection. You could start Dr. Blank on it when you return for your six month's checkup, and either just continue your present monthly amount for an extra month or so, or we could set up a new budget plan for you at that time with smaller monthly payments.

"As a matter of fact, I'm sure the doctor would agree that it would be a beautiful program to establish for the future. That is, plan on upgrading your entire mouth, say, one tooth at a time. This way you get one tooth restored, pay for it, get another one restored, pay for it, etc., until your total mouth is rebuilt."

This way your patient gets Plan I, or Plan II now, but will work toward Plan III on a gradual basis. Thus, having a goal, the patient has more reason to strive for his good dental health. It therefore becomes easier to keep him enthused about his teeth, and you have a better patient as well as a better referral service.

The Best Words Mean a Lot

Just like the familiar saying: "Little things mean a lot," the same applies to the language you use. Just the slightest hint of the right word or the wrong word can create a complete change of heart in a patient. Things can be running along perfectly smoothly until you or the dentist just happens to slip and say the wrong word or phrase completely unthinking, and the patient becomes sour, apprehensive, and may even decide to forego the entire proposed treatment. Contrariwise, you may find a patient very unimpressed and passive with the entire presentation. You can often say just the right thing at the right time to get the very proper response and full acceptance of the proposed case.

You, as well as the dentist, must always guard against that slip of the tongue—no matter how insignificant it may seem to you. For instance, it is just nothing at all for you and the doctor and other DAs to sit around talking about the amount of bleeding some extraction covered, or how much pain some toothache caused that patient the other day, or what a severe case of trenchmouth somebody had. Frankly, we all get so accustomed to these types of things that we easily forget that the patients are not hardened to terminology and can easily become alarmed at overhearing such talk. Don't ever slip and say the wrong thing within earshot of a patient.

On the other hand, always say the right things to your patients. If there is anything the patients need at case presentation, it's reassurance and confidence that they're making the correct decision and doing the right thing. This is where you come in. As mentioned earlier in this chapter, you the dental secretary, are in the unique position to insert just that correct word or phrase to put your patient at ease.

You know the words: discomfort, not pain; anesthetic, not injection or shot; efficient instead of quick; remove instead of extract or pull; prepare or reduce instead of grind down.

What about the other words? Convenient payments instead of budget payments; initial payment instead of down payment;

prepaid, instead of cash in advance; payment plan instead of contract.

You will, of course, have your own grouping of words and terminology in your own office and area, but my point is this: always think of the connotation a word or phrase might have to the lay person before you use it. Generally, you are strictly after the good thought waves—not the poor ones. Once you have adopted the most frequently used phraseology in your office, the everyday use of it will become second nature with you.

If you are sitting in on a conference between the doctor and the patient, you may find it convenient (unobtrusively) to interpret a point or two about a patient you recently had who had been treated in a similar fashion, and the excellent results the doctor attained there. Another good idea would be something like this: The dentist has just finished explaining to the lady patient that her anteriors should receive jackets for strength and protection. Now you can easily jump into the conversation with the exhilarated comment of how truly beautiful her smile would be if she had the jackets! Or, how lovely, or how very feminine. The patient is a man? How handsome, how manly, how masculine, how virile!

Note this: Words create visual pictures in our minds. If you want to make a pleasant impression on someone, you need only to create a beautiful mind picture or visualization, and you can do this with the correct words.

If I say, "ancient man," you immediately think of an old, old man bent over a cane, with his clothes hanging sloppily around him. His face is very wrinkled, his skin just hanging.

If I say "lovely lass," you usually think of a pert young lady, blond or red-haired, perhaps freckles, literally beaming with a smile and vitality.

Nice words make you feel good because of the image you paint yourself. Your task is to learn to help all of your doctor's patients to paint beautiful pictures in their minds about their dental health. In this way they will become far better patients, and will not only appreciate the work the doctor does for them, but they will care enough to take care of it. You will be much more likely to create dental missionaries instead of just satisfied patients.

9 | Teamwork: The Key to Success in Dentistry

Why You Were Hired

When you first came to work the chances were that neither you nor your employer knew much about each other. Sure, you had an interview or even two or three prior to your being hired, but you realize by now certainly that you really hardly knew each other. Basically you went to work here because you felt you would be able to fit in and could enjoy the practice and earn a suitable income. Likewise your dentist hired you because he felt you would be a valuable addition to his staff. He felt you were intelligent, honest, and hard working. He felt you either had skills or were capable of acquiring such skills as to become a real asset to the office. In addition, and very important, he felt you could fit into the team already established in the office.

Why Bother with Teamwork?

One might ask what is so important about teamwork. If each member of the staff is fully competent in his respective field and duties, it doesn't really matter and it is really rather unnecessary to help someone else with their chores—right? Wrong! The basic meaning of "teamwork" is to be unselfish. You must think and live teamwork and unselfishness hour after hour, day after day.

If you do try very hard to fit in and really become an integral part of the team, then it will soon become quite obvious to all of the others that you are trying, and they will almost automatically respond in kind. This is what the real meaning of teamwork implies. There is an old Indian term called "Potlatch." It basically means, "I will do more for you than you can do more for me." This epitomizes the basic spirit of the team approach. If all members of the team practice this, then you will all knit into a togetherness that cannot be beat. You will learn to anticipate each other's moves, reactions and desires so much that you will react accordingly in the best, most reinforcing manner to create a smooth running, "well-oiled" machine. This must be your goal, and the goal of each and every team member.

On the other hand, if each one of you feels as though the other team members must continually help you, then you yourself are the least desirable member. So, paraphrasing the late John F. Kennedy, "Think not of what the team can do for you, but of what you can do for the team."

Naturally, there are frequent tasks and chores that require that you call for assistance. This happens continually in the busy dental practice. And do not hesitate to call on another team member for help if you really need it, but make sure you honestly do find yourself unable to carry the burden without aid. Your teammate will not object if it is obvious her help is needed.

Contrariwise, it will be most gracious of you to be ever on the lookout for some way in which you can help your colleagues. Remember not to let your own duties lapse on a continual basis though. You will not be much of a teammate if you continuously let your own work slide in order to help someone else, and then have to have help in order to catch up again. If either of you sees this situation developing, you must take immediate steps to correct the situation. Sit down together at your first opportunity and discuss it frankly. Mutually decide from the team approach just how to get all the tasks completed in the most efficient manner. This is where the basic or "true grit" of the spirit of teamwork arises. It is working together on a particular problem; noting each other's problems, opinions, and assets, and blending them all for the perfect solutions.

On Getting Along with Others

As has been mentioned before, life in a close organization like a dental practice can get rather tense at times. It is all too easy for the personnel to get on one another's nerves. This is a normal reaction due to the heavy stresses of a busy practice, but it is not a normal reaction to let these petty stresses get out of hand. Sometimes it is only a tiny thoughtless comment made under pressure that can build slowly and continuously into a huge chasm that can split a team apart. This cannot ever be permitted to happen.

Sometimes it seems as though the entire office staff is on your back about something and it may not even be your fault! What should you do? The best solution for all concerned in the practice is to first make certain you are not at fault. If you are, then take immediate steps to correct the trouble. If, on the other hand, you are entirely blameless, go ahead and fix the solution as much as you can with little complaint, and then when the big trouble has blown over, and everyone is once again quiet and on an even temper, you can calmly and quietly explain your position to everyone. It would be best if you can more or less call a formal office conference for this presentation of your viewpoint. It is much more likely to be taken serious this way, and you can direct your remarks to the total staff. If you happen to talk to each staff member separately, then someone may easily misinterpret the tone of your voice or some specific wording and take offense to your remarks. Certainly any misinterpretation of your remarks at this point could only create more friction and hurt feelings.

How to Handle the Other Bosses

Frequently you will be in an organization that seemingly has nothing but bosses. Too many chiefs and not enough Indians, don't you know! It seems as though everyone wants to be the top dog and acts as if you are actually working for him. This can become quite disconcerting. You were hired for a rather specific job, with basically one employee, and yet other people keep giving you orders (or try to). You can go on and follow everyone's orders, and be subservient to all if you want to live that way, but frankly it doesn't make for very good teamwork. Teamwork is for all to more or less carry an equal load, and to help each other. If you are continually trying to carry someone else's load as well as your own, you will soon run out of steam and not be able to carry on your assigned duties. Likewise your attitude is bound to become rather bitter after a while. Looking at it another way, if the other auxiliary continually gets away with burdening you with some of her chores, her laziness is soon to become rather obnoxious, and basic resentment will be the inevitable result.

Now if you want to be the proper team member, you should politely sit down with the offending party and express your observations and feelings. Do not let it come down to personality differences if there is any possible way to avoid it. Whether you or the other employees like it or not, you have been hired to work together. If you wish to retain your employment at any dental office, you must get along with your fellow auxiliaries. Any dissension will show through and become obvious in your day-to-day working.

You must point out in a frank, but definitely pleasant manner to your bossy fellow employee that you feel you are being taken advantage of and declare specifically in which ways you feel you are being unfairly used. Be careful to maintain a level of self-control and permit no emotionalism to enter the picture. This is simply a straightforward, matter-of-fact type discussion of your viewpoint.

Then give the other party time for rebuttal, if any. This is mandatory for, after all, she has fifty percent of the rights, too. It could well be that she was completely unaware of the fact that she has been stepping on your toes. Let her answer step-by-step all of your complaints. Then the two of you can (hopefully) calmly work out whatever compromises are needed to even things out. Remember this important point—since you started this important conference, it becomes your task to keep it on an even keel and to permit no tempers to be lost. If any serious anger evolves from this meeting, you will likely find things even worse than before.

Note this: As I have mentioned above, it is possible that the other party was not even aware of stepping on your toes and "bossing" you. Some people simply have domineering personalities and do not realize it. When you point out something like this to them, you are in effect insulting them, and as this puts many people on the defensive, there is a tendency to strike back much harder than they would ordinarily. So keep it calm, cool and collected. Declare your views simply and to the point and try your very best to smooth things over to mutual advantage.

If you do not succeed this first time, wait a week or so and try again. This time you can be somewhat more forceful and to the point, since it will be obvious to your domineering colleague what you want.

If you get results now, work as smoothly with her as possible, even going out of your way to help her with some of her other chores (not the ones you've been doing for her). She will likely be undergoing some belittling and possibly degrading (to her) changes and the more reinforcement you can give her the better.

Please do not go too far, and become bossy yourself. This could be just as disastrous or more so. And just make absolutely certain that you are in the right. Give yourself a little self-appraisal before you accuse someone else. This way you are unlikely to become embarrassed for false accusations.

Now what if your conferences produce no results? You should then go to your employer and present the total facts to him as you see them. This then places the problem in his lap, and his handling of such may not suit you, so be well prepared to accept his decision pro or con.

If he decides for you, again go out of your way to help your antagonist overcome her defensive feelings. You must both work toward fairness and teamwork, as this is why you were hired.

If your dentist decides against you, then either resign or accept the talk with a good spirit. If you find you cannot continue your work without animosity, then you will be unable to carry your normal level of teamwork and you will be doing the best service to the office to resign.

What should you do if the other boss is the dentist's wife? This frequently becomes a rather touchy situation. You should never, never risk any sort of run-in with the doctor's wife. This cannot possibly end in anything satisfactory. If you offend her in any way you are just begging for trouble. It may be that you are completely without fault, but it is out of your hands. If she feels you are unsatisfactory for the office or has any gripes about your work in any way, you have very little recourse. She can complain enough to her husband, the dentist, that he has a choice put before him of either you go or she does—and you already know the answer to that decision.

So what to do if the dentist's wife demands too much of you? Try once (only) to suggest to her that you have been assigned other tasks by the doctor, and that you really have very little time to help her now. If she insists, you must drop what you are doing and follow her requests.

If it becomes a habit and you are unable to regularly complete your tasks, have a sincere, but friendly conference with your doctor and tell him you are unable to complete your normal duties *and* help his wife. Ask him *which* he would prefer be done. This will get you off the hook and relieve you of the burden of trying to do both. By taking the situation in your own hands this way you will be in a much better position to have your viewpoint listened to and accepted than if you let your office work slide until such a point that the dentist has to speak to you about it.

If you work in an office with two or more dentists, you'd better get it clarified right away to whom you are to answer. If each doctor feels you must do his bidding, you will most surely be caught in a totally impossible situation. Go to the dentist who originally hired you and point out the need to him for clarification of your work load. One person simply cannot work for two bosses unless there is a specifically spelled-out work order. Just do not specifically offend one of the employers by saying to him "No, I won't do it"; or "I don't have time." Something much less offensive will be better. Say, "May I finish this task for Dr. Jones first?" or something like, "Dr. Jones asked me to do this now, but I'll be glad to help you as soon as I finish. Is that all right with you?" Naturally if he insists, go ahead and help him, uncomplainingly, but call for your doctor-assistant conference later in order to correct the situation.

Does Rank Have Its Privileges?

This is a question that arises in nearly every dental practice at one time or another. At times it seems to reach tremendous proportions, but should never be permitted to become a consideration at all. In short, rank does not have its privileges in the dental team. Any insinuation that one member holds rank over another will be quite detrimental. It will break up a team sooner than almost anything else.

Unfortunately the potential exists all the time. Any time one member of the group has been employed longer than another, there is a tendency for two things to happen. First, the member of the staff who has been employed there for the longest time will frequently have to help in the office training of the new girl. This in itself tends to make her somewhat "bossy" if she is not readily cognizant of the fact that she is only helping out the team. If this task falls in your lap, always remember that while you have been around a while, you are expected to help the new girl until she can carry her own load, but after that point, your commanding, directing, and showing action must drop off to such a point as to be equalized within the team.

On the other hand, if you are the new girl in a team and must be dependent on your fellow auxiliary for directions, it behooves you to assert yourself when you gain enough knowledge, so that your colleague with seniority can know clearly that you need less help. In other words, if you continually have to ask for help and advice of the rest of the staff, you will have a tendency to create the "bossy" attitude unconsciously in the other individual.

So you see seniority means that you have been there a longer time, but not that you are privileged to hold this knowledge over your fellow auxiliaries.

If your office has a so-called office manager, make absolutely sure all of your duties and those of your other team members are clearly spelled (or written) out. If one member of the office staff has defined supervisory duties, you must know this in advance. You must know just how far these duties go and exactly which orders you are to follow and when. Be adamant about getting all of these points squared away in the beginning of your employment and you'll find the work will go much more smoothly and the teamwork will run perfectly.

So You Are Unhappy

After you have been working in a dental office for a number of months and are pretty knowledgeable about your work, and you suddenly take stock of yourself and feel that you are not enjoying your work, what should you do? I hope you will not just resign abruptly. This would be a wasteful thing after all the time and effort you have put in, and certainly wasteful of the doctor's time and money. The answer is to try to correct the situation to a point where you are happy, if possible.

First, sit down some quiet evening or even lunch time, when no one else is around to disturb you, and one-by-one write down on paper all of the things you can think of that make you dislike your work. Make sure you record every single item—no matter how insignificant it may seem. Sometimes it is the total sum of many little things that create the most trouble.

Next, set the paper aside for one week and do not look at it at all. Try not to even think about the items you have recorded.

Then after this seven-day period, get out the paper and reread all of the items on it. Do you still feel they are all true problems? Do you want to add any more? What you really need to do now is a little self-appraisal. Take each item separately and decide what your ideal solution to it would be. In doing this, ignore any potential obstacles—just put down the solution to each item that will correct it to its maximum. Finished?

Now, place yourself in your fellow dental assistants' place and see how many solutions will create problems for them. If you could correct problem one, would it make trouble for DA #1 or DA #2? If your ideal solution will create trouble for someone else, it just will not work, will it? So therefore devise some sort of compromise that will give you maximum results and yet be satisfactory (as far as you can tell) to your team members. This now becomes your new ideal correction. If you feel you cannot live happily with this compromise, continue to ponder it until you can arrive at something with which you can find contentment with as little potential problem for your colleagues as possible.

After you have done this with all the items on your list, again lay it aside for a week. Then go back to it and reread to be certain that if all the corrections were made according to your preferences (as compromised) you would be contented in your work. If something still bugs you, try to work it out so you can satisfy your conscience that you will not offend anyone seriously but yet attain happiness.

Incidentally, the week waiting periods are to give you a chance to cool off and possibly change moods. Sometimes we tend to overdo our gripes if we are in a foul mood, whereas we can be much more forgiving if we are in a pleasant frame of mind. The time periods are to try to give you the opportunity to review the gripes in various moods. On second glance you may even feel rather silly about putting down some of the items the first time. Contrariwise you may have first overlooked some important little gripe because it seemed rather trivial out of its normal context.

Once you have finally decided you have the best possible solutions to all of your problems, take them to your doctor for a personal conference. Present them to him with enough background information so that he knows you have worked hard in preparing them. Keep the entire presentation in its proper, level-toned perspective. Any emotional display could play havoc with what you are trying to do at this point. Tell the dentist simply and straightforward the problems as you see them and tell him why they make you unhappy. Then tell him what you have considered to be the best solution. Then stop talking.

Now his response at this point may not be exactly what you want, but don't worry too much if you get no definitive answer at all. Remember, you have spent two or three weeks on this, and have most likely caught him completely unawares. You do not want to back him into a corner or you may get the entire thing thrown back in your face (figuratively!), so you should suggest that you realize he needs some time to study your proposals, so would he please give you his response by, say, the middle of next week? You should not apply any pressure now, because again, you want him to analyze the work with an unbiased, unoffended frame of mind. Your total approval must be for him to see clearly your viewpoint. If you taint his opinion now, you can consider your cause lost.

After he has had an opportunity to adequately look at the situation (he may wish a few days to observe the actions of the office in motion), the two of you can then sit down again and hash out the difficulties. He can go along with you totally, or partially, or not at all. You can then decide what you wish to do.

If you get no affirmative response at all, you can resign if you feel you simply cannot continue working under these conditions. If, however, you feel that time may possibly alter the situation or you feel you can live with the problems, just continue to do your best every day and don't work with a constant chip on your shoulder. This sour attitude could get you discharged and you do not want that on your record.

If your doctor rejects all points, or major ones, ask him if he has any objections to your discussing the situation with your other team members. Here you may not do anything that would be contrary to his desires for the office. You must not ever create any inkling of undermining of his authority. The old axiom must apply here, "He may not always be right, but he is always boss." The only situations you should freely discuss with the other assistants would be friction between you and them personally. Never talk about your disagreements with your employer with other auxiliaries. This will only serve to lower your esteem in the eyes of the team.

If some solutions singly don't seem to get ironed out between you and the doctor, or you and the other assistants, and you feel it may help, call for a general office conference and air the complaint here. Get your doctor's okay on this first, as you do not want to embarrass him or create an affront to him. In this way you can frequently get results by using three, four or five or more minds working together instead of just one or two. The other girls may not realize your viewpoint and may be able to offer a simple solution.

Remember that happiness is a state of mind. Do not expect the world to lie down at your feet, and do not expect supreme happiness at all times. Also, don't forget that other people have problems too and that in the close-knit workings of the dental office, there must be continual give and take. It is a marriage of several minds working toward the one goal—better dentistry. Always keep this goal in mind and you will frequently find your individual problems will diminish greatly. And you can continue to work toward becoming the world's greatest Dental Assistant.

part 2

The Chairside
Assistant

10 *How to Master Patient Control*

Techniques of Getting the Patient to Relax

Probably the real key to the successful day in the dental office is to have easy patients upon which to work. What a happy time it is when you find you have a real friend in the chair. He is pleasant, congenial, communicates well, cooperates. He opens wide and generally relaxes so that your doctor and you can get on with the work at hand. Just seeing on the morning schedule that Mr. Niceguy is coming seems to cheer up the entire staff.

What makes him so nice? He is relaxed. He has total confidence in the dental team's abilities to do the job, and he has been made physically comfortable.

It therefore behooves you, the DA, to make a maximum effort to literally train each patient to relax in the chair, and thus become a better patient.

Let's start at the beginning. By the time the patient arrives at the door of the treatment room, we will assume the dental secretary has already done her share of the relaxation program. He has been greeted pleasantly, had coffee offered, had a few moments to sit in a pleasant reception room with background music, and up-to-date readable magazines. He has been told how long he will have to wait, so he will not become apprehensive about that. He has probably had some pleasant, distracting small talk with the dental secretary, so he has had little time to sit and worry about his impending treatments.

Now he is ushered into the treatment room and he must notice as few "terrible-looking tools" as possible. If at all possible, the dental secretary brings the patient to the door of the operatory and he is there met with a cheery smile on your face.

All possible instruments are covered—especially the anesthetic syringe. It is usually quite convenient to simply cover the instrument tray or bracket table with the bib that will be placed around his neck. If your dentist practices upright dentistry and the patient must sit up and look at the bracket tray full of instruments, at least keep the bib over them until the dentist is about ready to start. If the patient will be expected to wait in the chair for several minutes before the doctor arrives, it certainly isn't very relaxing to spend the time peering at a bunch of sharp-looking tools.

Keep that needle cover on! Most people have difficulty becoming truly relaxed when they are forced to stare at an open syringe and needle—with possibly a drop of solution hanging off the point.

Swing the instrument tray or bracket table as far away from the patient's view as possible. For the sake of efficiency you should go ahead and insert the burs you anticipate will be needed by the doctor, but try to swing the handpieces away also.

If your dentist practices sitting down you should proceed to tilt the chair back as soon as is practical. Men may wish to loosen their ties and shirt collars and ladies may wish to rearrange their skirts, so permit ample time for this. If possible you should have a definite place for patient's purses, packages, glasses, etc. In the average office, a small triangular shelf in a corner works beautifully. If should ideally be placed in such a position as to permit the patient to see it. Occasionally we happen to have some of those suspicious souls who feel that you might search through their purse while they are in the chair. If they can see it at all times they will have a tendency to relax more.

If you adjust the chair and the patient for the doctor, you

should say something, pleasant to him to the effect: "The doctor will want to treat you in this position, is this comfortable enough for you?" In this way you have let them realize they must more or less accept this position for treatment by the dentist, but it also tells them you are interested in their comfort.

If you anticipate from the patient's reaction, temperament, and conversation that he is literally scared to death, you must immediately try to take his mind off of his fears and console him. This applies to any age or sex, of course.

Ask leading questions of the patient. That is, ask him (or her) questions that he must think to answer, and that cannot be answered with yes or no. Now don't ask, "How are you today?" A "fine," or an "okay," or similar will do little to take his mind off of his fears. Ask something like, "What kinds of flowers do you have planted in your garden?" (He must now think enough to enumerate the various types.) Or, "What have the children (grandchildren) done lately?" or "What do you think the President should do about ————?" The key here is to try to ascertain some interests of the patient. It is usually a much better time to do this friendly, informal questioning on the patient's first visit or two, prior to his having any serious treatment. Usually if a person knows there is to be very little treatment or uncomfortable (painful) work done, he is likely to be much more talkative and you, the secretary, the hygienist or the doctor should make a brief one-word note on the patient's chart just what subject or things the patient likes.

For instance, if the patient seems to like to discuss his grandchildren, write down "grandchildren" on his chart. Then anyone or specifically you can easily recall this fact when you see him again and ask him to tell you some interesting things they have done lately. If you have the opportunity and care to be somewhat more specific, you may care to jot down "grand-children—2g, 4b," which of course means two girls and four boys.

Or the patient may like to discuss "gardening," or "sewing," or "dogs," or "cats," or "cars," "boats," "planes," "camping," or "camper" (if he has a mobile camper and takes trips as compared to "camping" which may be more confined to summer season), "fishing," "painting," "crafts," "photography." I could go on and on, but you can certainly grasp the meaning. Keep your note-word short because you will usually have very little time to write more than a word or so.

On subsequent notes you may wish to add other note-words as you and the patient discuss other subjects. You will not necessarily need to keep a record of every subject covered, of course, because you will no doubt have many similar conversations with different patients all during the week—just keep a note on the ones that seem to have more importance, and bring forth more response from the patient.

A word on conversation with the patient: try your dead level best to keep it under control so you can bring it to an abrupt halt if you are called away from the chair. If the patient is in total command of the conversation, you will not be able to leave without possibly offending him, and that's not good.

If you find that some specific subject is getting out of hand, that is, the patient is putting you on the defensive, or is discussing a very touchy subject (sex, religion, gossip, etc.), you must excuse yourself graciously, look at your watch, and "remember" that you suddenly need to check on those X-rays, (or the sterilizer), or ask the patient another leading question about some other subject. Do not ever permit any of the taboo subjects to come into a conversational framework in the office. It will do no one any good at all and could do a lot of damage if it got around that your office was having discussions on politics, religion, sex or most particularly gossip about some specific individuals.

Let's face it, sometimes your doctor will enter into some taboo talks with some specific patients from time to time. He shouldn't, and he probably knows this, but after all it's his practice and he can do what he darn well pleases—even if he could hurt his reputation and lose patients this way.

On Anticipating the Doctor

When the dentist is operating, it is your duty to help him in every conceivable manner, and this goes beyond routine chairside assisting. Remember that he is carrying a tremendous amount of tension and responsibility. He is responsible for the accuracy of his diagnosis and must follow through with vital accuracy through his hands. Any relief of his tension you can give him will certainly be appreciated. So do your very best to relieve him of all possible chores and anticipate his every move.

You should do this by first learning all of his systematic approaches to each service he renders. That is, if he is doing an amalgam restoration, he will probably follow a certain predetermined pattern of attack. It may go something like this: He may start with a #557 bur in the high speed handpiece. Then, following that, he may switch to a round bur in the slow speed handpiece. He may follow this with a spoon excavator, then go to a chisel or hatchet, then be ready for a specific base or liner and proceed to the matrix. In packing the restoration, he may always start with a specific amalgam plugger, say a #1, after about three applications of amalgam from the amalgam carrier, he may wish to switch to a #2, 3 or 5 or 6 plugger, or to an overcondenser of some sort. Then, in carving, he may always begin with an explorer, then go to a specific favorite carver.

Now you can certainly realize that each dentist will have his own specific procedures for all his services. And unfortunately for you, your doctor may not use any specific time-after-time pattern. If this is the case, you would do well to point out to him in a friendly manner that if he can follow a specific pattern (at least as much as possible) in every service he renders, you will be in a much better position to anticipate his needs and help him. The main point is, of course, that he can work more quickly, smoothly, and easily if you already have the next anticipated instrument waiting for him even before he asks for it. And he will most certainly work more relaxed if he knows you will have it waiting for him. You simply save him one more decision, or one more command or request. By the end of the day a few such savings can change one's entire physical and emotional being. He can even go home almost relaxed instead of grouchy.

So make it your business from now on to learn all you can about your doctor's needs at the chair. If he isn't certain, you can do very little to help, but you should encourage him as politely as possible to streamline his own techniques.

This streamlining has a basic philosophy at its core: never use the same instruments twice. This means always completely finish with an instrument before you (the doctor) discard it. If he uses a 557, then a spoon, then a 557 then a #6, then a 557, he is practicing very inefficiently. He should look ahead during the preparation sufficiently to anticipate all of the necessary usage of the 557, before laying it aside. And he should not find it necessary to use it again once it has been laid aside.

Naturally you must not tell your doctor how to do his work so blatantly, but you can conveniently mention that you were reading in "this book" or "that journal" the other night how following this procedure could reduce effort and time, too. (He may be impressed that you are interested enough in your profession that you do reading after hours!) In this way you might persuade him to better his techniques without stepping on his authoritative toes and hurting his feelings. You must not leave him with the impression that you feel he is behind the times. If, however, you can gently move him to a more specific procedure on one individual task, you can more easily prod him to all others, and the truth is you can soon become that "well-oiled machine" you should be.

How to Control the Talkative Patient

One of the more worrisome problems that you have is the talkative patient. You know him, the one who continually makes attempts at conversation—with anyone who will listen. The basic reason for his action is insecurity about the impending dentistry, but this patient simply must be controlled if your doctor is to have any successful production at all. As is the case all too frequently in the dental office, it becomes the chore of the chairside assistant to control this patient. If the patient should take any offense to anyone in the office, it is always better if it is not the doctor. After all, he is the last resort and if he has a patient who is unhappy with something about his (or her) dental treatment or personal treatment and the dentist desires to keep Mrs. Jones happy, he can always make a final attempt to smooth things over. If he has offended someone, there is simply no chance that you could help. After all, the patients come to see the dentist, not his assistants (usually!).

If the patient enters into a simple friendly conversation and you can anticipate brevity, then be friendly and let the conversation come to a pleasant close. If you have a few moments, it is certainly good public relations to chat with the patient. This will help put him at ease and make him more cooperative, as has been discussed earlier in this chapter.

So, if you find yourself with a talker or a mutterer, please make haste to take control of the situation.

This patient almost starts talking the moment he opens the front door, and just will not stop. It becomes quickly apparent that your doctor will be delayed by simply entering the room, because he cannot pop in and pop out without speaking to the patient and to walk away will offend him, so you must head this off.

As soon as you have the patient seated and ready for the doctor, tell the patient that the doctor is extremely busy today (not "rushed"–"busy") and will probably want to stop in for about one minute for the preliminaries and the anesthetic if needed, and then will need to leave again. Then you should leave and not give the patient an opportunity to tie you up in conversation. Tell the dentist what you have done so that he can follow through and not make it seem as though you are pulling a fast one.

If the patient ignores this hint and starts conversation with the dentist, you should do one of two things. Look at your watch. Try to make sure the patient can notice you checking it, but don't make a production of it or it will seem artificial. Then work your way into the conversation and tell the doctor he must tend to "that inlay" now, or must check "that X-ray film" now, or must check on the setting time of those models, or must run the slump test now, or some such nonsense as this. He can easily stop any conversation abruptly and dash out. If you wish, you can dash out too, excusing the two of you politely and telling the patient you'll be right back in a monent or so.

Something else you can try is to walk out while the doctor and the patient are talking, and while in another room ring the bell or buzzer system that the doctor (and the patient) will hear. The dentist can then make a small abrupt hesitation, and excuse himself. The patient will be led to believe the doctor was forced to leave when he'd really rather sit and chat with him.

Another trick is fine if you have two phone lines. Either you or the secretary can call in on the other line (this is fine as long as the telephone ring can be heard by the patient), and the doctor can be called to the telephone. If you have a telephone or intercom in the operatory, the doctor can easily be interrupted and called out.

Or, the secretary can simply walk in and stick a note under the doctor's nose so to speak. The doctor will read it, (the patient cannot see it) and abruptly excuse himself. The note may have absolutely nothing written on it, or the secretary may write some suitable word on it, as she wishes. The point is the patient will believe the "note" was important and the doctor had to leave when he'd really rather remain. Naturally, you'd better make certain the dentist is well aware of your tactics, otherwise you'd have a very embarrassing time on your hands, trying to explain to the doctor in front of the patient why you're trying to get him out of the room.

If the patient tries to talk as the dentist is trying to get started on the treatment, put a saliva ejector in his mouth. This will slow many patients down. Then, if necessary, add a cotton roll or two or three.

If the patient seems to be in some sort of real distress, you might just have to remove everything from his mouth and let him tell you his problem. But if you see this was just an excuse to slow down the work, pop it all back in as soon as you can.

Sometimes the patient will not stop a conversation long enough for you to even get a saliva ejector in, so you should gently place your finger on his forehead and ease his head back into the headrest (if not already there) and place the saliva ejector tip to his lips and saying nothing, work in in, even though he is still trying to talk. You can do the same with a cheek retractor or a mouth mirror.

If he still continues to try to talk, your last resort is to simply place your hand on his shoulder to get his attention, and interrupt him and say, "Mr. Jones, if the doctor is to treat your tooth, (teeth, mouth, gums) properly for you today, you'll simply have to stop talking and let us continue with the treatment." This may offend him so be sure to have a sincere, honest smile and tone of voice when you say it.

If he ceases, then everything is fine. But if he should start up again in a few minutes, you should again tap him on the shoulder gently and "shush" him. If absolutely no resorts are left, you should tell him to "please be quiet."

If none of the above have worked, then it is finally up to your doctor to make the next decision. He may accept it and treat the patient that way, or he may wish to discharge him from the office for the day or the practice totally.

Remember that more than likely the patient is very nervous and afraid. It may help if the doctor gives the patient some preoperative sedation or tranquilizer. If it is not important (to the doctor), the patient may wish to try a second appointment this way in preference to booting him out. Or he may wish to elevate his fees to this patient to compensate for the additional time required for treatment. One thing is for certain, few dentists can afford many patients like this.

How to Soothe the Disturbed or Boisterous Patient

Occasionally you will run into someone who is mentally or emotionally ill. These people can present real difficulty for control, and it is impossible to adhere to any one or two set rules or patterns for control. Each patient may need to be handled on an individual basis. In fact it may frequently be necessary to use multiple techniques on a single patient at the same appointment.

Point number one is to try to learn as much background information as possible about this patient. He has probably been under someone's care for some time and you or the secretary should first speak to this custodian. Ask how the custodian controls the patient under various circumstances. Find out the patient's response to these various control measures. Call the patient's physician (or ask the secretary to call) and get his advice. Then, armed with all of this information, tell your dentist what you have learned and he can act accordingly. Naturally, he can call these people, but if you or the dental secretary do it for him and as completely as he would wish, he will appreciate your efforts and realize that you have saved him time.

Incidentally, it is frequently a good help to sedate these ill patients, but your doctor will always want you to have checked with the patient's physician. Whenever you call the M.D., remember that he, too, is a very busy man. Call the physician's secretary or nurse and do this: tell her who you are (Dr. Smith's assistant), that the dentist will need to perform certain procedures on the patient (fillings or periodontal treatments, or extraction or whatever), and you expect it to require so many appointments lasting for so many minutes each and over so many weeks. The dentist expects to need to use local anesthetic a number of times. Would she be so kind as to ask the physician if he has any recommended preoperative sedation or precautions. Otherwise, the dentist will make his own choices.

The important thing here is to save both yourself and the physician's office time. Know in advance what you need to say for background information, relate it precisely to the M.D.'s nurse and be prepared to receive precise information back in return.

If by some chance the patient has been relatively quiet and in the middle of treatment suddenly decides to react in a boisterous manner, you must quickly help the dentist control the situation. The patient may grab the doctor's arm or hand. He may jerk his head, or may well make an attempt to climb out of the chair. Try diligently to anticipate the doctor's wishes here. If necessary hold and restrain the patient's arms or head as much as possible. Keep instruments out of obvious reach of the patient if possible. If necessary buzz for the secretary or rover to come in and assist in the restraint.

All the while try to get through to the patient (with as much of a sincere and pleasant smile you can muster) that you do want to help him. The dentist will certainly be doing the same, and your actions can reinforce his. You should not raise your voice or frown at the patient as this may disturb him even more. Psychologically it frequently helps the patient to know he has a "friend" (you) there while he is undergoing all that turmoil by the enemy (the dentist) whom he may well depict as not liking him. If you can see this type of reaction, try to emphasize to him your wishes to be his friend and sort of exude—even overdo—sincere concern, friendship, and sympathy. Try to distract him from his fears. The doctor will certainly not mind the patient's liking you more and will appreciate it if he can get on with his treatment.

If the patient starts screaming or cursing, you should quickly try to get the door closed to muffle the noise. Even if there are no other patients in the office at the time, the telephone may ring and to have someone call for an appointment and hear screams in the background is not too desirable, is it? Buzz for the secretary to close the door if you cannot get away yourself.

If the patient curses you or the dentist, just ignore everything he says. Keep remembering that he is ill and upset, and is really not directing his venom at you as a person, but rather as a figure of authority. You may ask the patient to be quiet or to stop using foul language, but the chances are he will continue just to spite you. At any rate, you can ask him firmly once and if that is to no avail, don't bother asking again. If you can anticipate that your presence disturbs the patient, it may be best if you leave the treatment room completely. Don't do this, of course, without asking the doctor first.

Remember that a patient with this emotional or mental instability can have very rapid mood changes. Because of this, you may find yourself with a screaming, yelling, rowdy patient one moment, and then, lo, a few moments later this same patient may be quite sedate and as fine and cooperative a patient as you could ask for, and the next moment, he may be boisterous again. Be fully prepared to react to his varied moods just as promptly as he changes them.

The Angry Patient

Occasionally we all get hold of the angry patient. This is the man or woman who is very unhappy with something you or the doctor has done "to" her (as compared to "for" her). She is here today to get it corrected or know the reason why, and you'd just better believe that she'll tell the whole world about her unhappiness if it's not corrected.

Since it probably is the doctor who is getting the brunt of her tirades, you, the chairside assistant can be in a unique position to help smooth things over, and calm her down. Usually the dental secretary will have some prior hint to give you that she's angry—hence the appointment—and it is usually best if you can intercept this patient in the chair before she gets to see the doctor.

It might be added here that it's best if she can tell her problem to the dental secretary first—completely—before you see her. Then ask her to tell it *completely* to you. And after a while, she'll have to tell it completely again to the doctor. The purpose of this is that each time she tells it, she will lose a little of her steam and anger, and hopefully, by the time the doctor sees her, she will be considerably cooler in temperament.

But before you call in the dentist, and after she has told her story to you, you should do everything you can to answer her complaints. Be truthful and straightforward—any dodging will be quickly picked up by the patient, and this will only make matters worse. Give her the kind of answers you feel the doctor would give. Never side against the dentist! If you feel she has a legitimate gripe against him, and if you can think of no back-up for him, say nothing at all.

But you should give Mrs. Angry Lady all the reassurance possible. If you can determine it as a case of faulty dentistry you can explain that if the doctor finds he has done something wrong, he will gladly correct it. (Do not emphasize *if* to the patient.) It is just a fact of life that we are all human and subject to mistakes, and if the dentist makes an error, he will want to correct it.

Most frequently the problem will lie in poor communications. Either she has overestimated the expected result or she was not clearly made knowledgeable of the possible deficiencies. You should do your best to answer her complaints for her before she sees the dentist. If her crown is sensitive, explain that practically all are sensitive for sometimes weeks or even months afterward, simply because of the fact that a tooth preparation is major surgery. After all, each tooth is an organ, and each time a bur or stone cuts a tooth, it is a surgical operation. It is hard tissue instead of soft, and a drill is used instead of a knife, but it is still an operation. The doctor placed "sufficient" (is "ample" a better term?) cement bases under it to compensate for the average tooth, but some teeth are just more sensitive than others following treatment. If it is too high, it is a simple matter of adjustment.

Occasionally teeth simply do not survive the operation—just like normal humans and general surgery. No tooth has a label on it declaring whether or not it will survive, but the death of a pulp as a result of the treatment is very, very rare. Anyway, these statements will give you some ideas as to how to respond to the patient's complaints.

If this doesn't satisfy her and/or the dentist still needs (or wants) to see her, go and call him. Tip him off first that she's angry about this or that so he will not be caught completely off guard. Then he will probably ask her to go over her complaints again. He will probably ask her, "Is there anything else?" after each pause in her story. In this way he will draw her out and it will tend to make her complaints (if they are not very legitimate) seem rather minimal to her. In fact, she will frequently have reached the point where her anger will be completely dissipated, and she will say something to the effect that "this last tooth you fixed is a little sensitive, but I gues it is not too bad. I just wanted you to check it." In this fashion, potential extreme difficulties can be drastically minimized.

The Proper Discharge

After your doctor finishes with his patient, it is usually your duty to make the final chair discharge. At this point you are in a unique position to reinforce the patient's confidence in the doctor and to help insure the patient's desire to be an even better patient next time.

You should remove the bib and return the chair to the best position for the patient to leave from. Be aware that completely upright may not necessarily be the best position for the patient to get up from.

Always check to insure that each and every patient has been properly cleaned up before letting them leave the treatment room. Look at them with the eye of the next patient sitting apprehensively out in the reception room. Is there any blood lingering on the patient's face? A moistened 2 x 2 sponge works well, as does a moistened facial tissue. (A tissue is cheaper, too.) Also wipe off any remaining amount of impression material.

Incidentally, something many patients appreciate is for the chairside assistant to squirt a little mouthwash around following treatment, and then you either suction it all out or let them empty their mouth in the basin. This leaves them with a somewhat better taste in their mouth.

Before this final discharge of the day, hand them their glasses. Try very hard to get an opportunity to clean their glasses for them. They will appreciate it.

Hand the ladies their purses, and other apparatus, and the men their coats if they are hung in the treatment room.

At this point, if the dentist expects it of you, go over any home care and postoperation instructions with them. If the dentist had already done this, at least repeat the main point or two for them. You can point out briefly any anticipated problems, such as cold sensitivity, waiting times prior to chewing, bleeding, pain, and such. It is always a good thing to emphasize that your doctor wants them to call him if there is any problem. Since you and he have carefully discussed all normal difficulties to be expected, such calls are quite rare, but it does give the patient peace of mind to know he can call and not disturb the dentist.

Whenever possible without seeming insincere, compliment the patient on his cooperation today. Naturally, you will look like an idiot if you said he was cooperative when you had to step on him a few times. But always try very hard to find some way to have some sort of compliment with which to say farewell to the patient, and be cheerful and smiling. Your most important point is to have the patient leave in as good a frame of mind as possible so he will have the fewest number of bad memories for his next trip here.

If you can get ample samples, or if you can get your doctor to furnish them, why not give the patients who have had heavy dentistry a couple of aspirins or the equivalent? Tell them to take them about the time they first begin to feel the local anesthetic leaving. They will appreciate your thoughtfulness.

While the Doctor Is Gone

In the average busy dental office, the doctor frequently comes in, maybe gives an injection, then leaves for a while to let the anesthetic take effect. Then, if you follow him, the patient is left alone with his fears and thoughts. And if he is at all inquisitive, he will look at the instruments if he can see any. All of this does very little to relax and soothe him.

Do this: always keep a supply of literature in the treatment room. If you both must leave, just hand the patient a magazine or book of jokes, or such.

If your doctor so desires, have a ready supply of dental patient education literature available instead, and give this to the patient. In this manner some constructive education of the patient can take place while you're gone. Some patients will frankly prefer casual literature, but most by far will read whatever you give them without complaint. It works especially well if you, knowing the patient is to receive, say, a fixed bridge, give him literature concerning bridges. The same with endodontia, periodontia, orthodontia, and so forth. Remember, the more dentally educated the patient, the better he will be and the more readily he will accept quality dentistry.

Some offices go so far as to provide audiovisual education during these few minutes. You can have your doctor make up a series of slides for information, with nothing more than a simple program such as a picture of a bridge, then a slide or two telling what it is, then another type of bridge, more descriptive slides and so on.

If you can anticipate a wait as long as eight to ten minutes, you can provide the patient with a regular filmstrip, record or tape showing on one of the Dukane projectors or new movie projectors.

A very simple, and extremely handy audiovisual is the General Electric "Show 'n Tell." It has a number of showings on various phases of dentistry, and the showings are brief—about three minutes.

A simpler setup, but one that works well for the patient, is the GAF viewer. It shows films and description of dentistry just by having some background light. The patient peers through it like the old stereoscopes.

If you are available to stay with the patient, you can pursue his dental education, too. Again, knowing he is to have a fixed bridge, you can tell him about the bridge—the various types—and what they do and don't do, and you could even show him some slides, too. Just hold them with your fingers with the ceiling light in the background, and the patient can get the picture.

In these days of preventive dentistry and with the emphasis on plaque control, you could easily work with the patient's home care procedures. Have him practice his flossing, or give him a sterilized toothbrush and let him show you his brushing method, to see if he needs help. This will help him, but it will also pass the time for you both in a profitable manner.

If permitted in your state, you could polish the patient's fillings. Also, if you are wandering around his mouth you could point out weak areas in his teeth with a hand mirror. These would be weakened cusps, chipped amalgam margins, fractured enamel, silicates beginning to wash out, plastics showing marginal leakage. Here the patient would actually see more of what the doctor sees, and would much more readily accept his diagnosis in the future, if you had already pointed out some of the areas to him. You could go so far as to point out that, for instance, in the case of that molar with the enormous old amalgam in it, that the doctor frequently has to place crowns there for best strength. He may need one some day, and now has already been told in advance to expect it. You have not made a diagnosis per se, just a declaration that many such teeth need this or that.

By constantly teaching, training, showing each patient more and more about his mouth, there will come a day when little time need by spent on convincing a patient to accept a diagnosis and treatment plan. Wouldn't your doctor appreciate that?

11 | *The Instrument Setup*

How to Obtain a More Efficient Procedure

One of the more important attributes of the quality chairside assistant is speed. If she is rapid, the doctor can be rapid in a corresponding manner. Therefore a major key to the maximum production of a dental team is the handling and manipulating of instruments.

As is usually the case, speed can be increased by better efficiency—and this in turn can be bettered by constant thought and preplanning.

The way to start is by first knowing what your doctor proposes to do on this patient or that. If you can know in advance you can get a head start on things and lay out many anticipated instruments ahead of time. Unfortunately it is frequently the case that the dentist doesn't know in advance just what he will be doing. In such instances, you should attempt to follow the motto of the Boy Scouts—"Be Prepared." In other words, be prepared for just about any procedure that may be called for. Know where every instrument is for every procedure. If the doctor is treating a specific problem, be prepared to suddenly switch to an entirely different task, and know where you can get every single instrument or piece of apparatus instantly. There should never be any extended waiting on the part of the dentist while his assistant goes to another room to hunt for a certain tool. Know your office so well that you could almost find every individual instrument in the dark.

Now in order to do this, you must follow the old adage, "A place for everything, and everything in its place." If you just lay sterilized instruments down in the nearest drawer, without any thought about next time, you may very well not remember next time where you placed them. Therefore, go through your entire office and systematically decide the best place for all instruments, then place them there.

Do not just lay them down in the order you found them, but have some specific order and regimentation to it. For instance, place the most frequently used instruments in the most easily accessible spot. Place the mouth mirrors and explorers in a drawer of the cabinet closest to the chair. Next, place the next most frequently used instruments beside these, and the next and so on. Since every dental office is different, you will need to work out your own specifics in your own office, but be sure to think it out carefully and plan it well. If you set it up once and change it the next week because it doesn't work, and the following week for the same reason, you've missed the point.

It may help you to lay it out on a paper sketch at first. This way you can mentally go through the various procedures of your office and see how it works. If you made a mistake, a simple erasure works fine. After following this technique several days, or even a week, you'll arrive at as close a solution as is possible. Don't be too alarmed if you make a few errors; just keep them minimized.

Don't forget to get your dentist's okay and advice on this. If you suddenly move every instrument without his prior knowledge, you may find yourself with a rather peculiar expression facing you.

If you have (all offices do) instruments or equipment or special cements that may only be used every few months, it frequently becomes rather difficult to recall instantly where it is kept. In this case, keep a neat typewritten list of every specific item you are concerned with, and list exactly where you are keeping it. You do not have to do this for the every day or even every week items, because you know them by heart, don't you? Make this list alphabetical, and allow about three spaces between lines, so you can add more from time to time and keep it alphabetical. If you need to, retype it for additional spacing and clarity. Have on it specifics such as, "copper cement powder and liquid–lab, second shelf, right"; "gold foil holder–storage room instrument tray, second tray from left"; "special shade guides– darkroom shelf." Your location notations need to be clear enough to direct anyone in the office to it, but brief enough to be uncluttering on the list. See Figure 11-1.

Adding machine paper—storage closet, top shelf, rear

Amalgam—lab, third open shelf on right

Anesthetic—lab, cabinet over sink, top shelf

Burs—white room, storage drawer

Cotton rolls—coral room, main storage cabinet, lower

Charts—business office, right cabinet, lower first shelf

Dycal—blue room, upper right cabinet, top shelf

Gold—lab, first shelf over casting machine

Light bulbs (ceiling)—storage closet, top shelf, rear

Light bulbs (unit)—lab, cabinet two, top shelf, center

Paper towels—storage closet, box on floor

Pencils—storage closet, second shelf, right

Saliva ejectors—lab, cabinet above sink, first shelf

Toilet paper—toilet, under sink

Typewriter paper—storage closet, second shelf, left

Wax (blue)—lab, second shelf over work bench

Wax (green)—coral room, storage cabinet, lower shelf

Wax (pink)—lab, cabinet three, first shelf on right

X-ray film—darkroom, side cabinet, first shelf

X-ray solutions—darkroom, lower cabinet, first shelf

Figure 11-1:   Supply List

If this listing is kept up-to-date, and in as close to alphabetical order as is possible, it is a very easy task to find any bulk stock in the entire office.

Keep the list on a clipboard in a convenient spot where the majority of your equipment is stored. It should not be in the treatment rooms, as it would be an unnecessary object to clutter it up. If you can arrange it in your office, have all such materials and instruments stored in one place or room, and have the list in plain view in that room. This way it will take no more than thirty seconds to get any instrument or supply in the entire office and production can continue at a rapid and efficient pace.

Don't forget that all X-ray supplies should ideally be stored in the darkroom. And also, you should keep a list of business office supplies and their location in a similar manner.

In order to work as an efficient team, both you and the dentist must have the same goals in mind. If you feel that you can streamline a procedure, tell him so, and why you think it will help and what he must do in order to help you; so the final result will be peak efficiency with minimal lost motion. What I am getting at here is that a dentist can frequently be the most inefficient piece of equipment in the office. Your major job may be to persuade him to alter his established techniques sufficiently so that you can help him better.

Inefficiency is doing something in more steps than necessary. Concentrate on this at all times. If your dentist uses a, say, #557, then a #6, then a #557 again, then a #4, or #6, then back to the #557, he is being inefficient. If he uses a hatchet, then a spoon, then the hatchet again, he is being inefficient. Both he and you must watch out for this sort of thing.

Let me say here in defense of the dentist that frequently the tooth demands inefficient treatment. There is just no way you can always avoid having to repeat the use of a tool, but you must continually try to think ahead enough to minimize it.

If a base is to be needed, the doctor should realize it very quickly in his preparation of the tooth and tell you then, so you can be getting out the cement, slab, spatula, etc. You should be all ready to mix it by the time he requests it. Frequently you can anticipate his moves so that you could begin your cement mix before he is ready for it and by good study and timing, both you and he would be ready simultaneously. That's efficiency.

He should concentrate on always starting similar procedures with the same instrument, and working systematically through a series. This way you can better anticipate his needs and have it ready for him before he needs it. (See chapter 10.)

In other words, in order to help him best, he must help you. You must be able to depend on him to follow closely an exactly predetermined method of treating a patient. If he is lackadaisical and sloppy about his tools, with little or no preset technique specifics, you can do little to help him efficiently. In effect, there will be no teamwork.

I would suggest that you sit down with him at an office conference and completely—and politely—discuss the situation. It may be that he simply does not know or realize your capabilities or the potential of the practice through proper utilization of your services. Remember, the vast majority of dentists today received their training prior to the days of four-handed dentistry and have never received formal (or even informal) training in auxiliary utilization. It is up to you to enlighten him. Please don't insult his intelligence—be tactful about it. Remember as always that each dentist is high on the mountain—he's the top dog and he is quite accustomed to making the decisions and directions. To interpret some conversation that emphasizes his ignorance or ineptitude will hardly please him, and you certainly will be able to continue in your job a lot longer with a boss who is not annoyed with you.

So sit down with him at a formal conference and point out to him—step-by-step—just how he can use you more effectively. Go over a recent case. Note to him how, if you had been properly utilized, he could have done so much more. Be specific. He would have had time to place four more surfaces of amalgam or two more silicates, or could have gone ahead with that sudden conversion from an alloy to a crown instead of having to place a temporary filling and reschedule. Point out that his productive income would have increased by $30, $40, or $50 (specifically), with very little increase in his labors. After all, it is you that is picking up the brunt of the work, not him.

If your doctor is the type who just likes to go at a slower pace, and really isn't that interested in making more money, show him (tell him) how much more of his work you can do for him if he will only let you. Then he will be able to leave the patient more frequently or sooner and go have a rest, a cigarette, cup of coffee, or whatever. You can make his life easier; his pace smoother.

If he is the sympathetic type, play on his sympathies and tell him how boring it is as a do-little dental assistant. Tell him you'd be so much happier as a full-service dental auxiliary. You'd rather be busy—steadily—than to dawdle and piddle around. Tell him that like the women's libbers, you feel unfulfilled.

Anyway, once you get him converted to your way of thinging, the two of you should go over step-by-step each major procedure. The two of you should plan just what *you* can do to help and what *he* should do to let you help more. Plan an upcoming case. After he decides where he will work on Mrs. Jones' next appointment, both of you "work through" the case, movement after movement. In doing this each one should decide exactly what each duty will be. Determine who will retract tongue or tissue and at what time during the procedure. Decide which burs will be most likely to be used and in what order. Then go to the hand instruments, in order, and then to which type of matrix retainer. Who shall set them up and who shall place them on the teeth? What should the assistant do while the dentist is busy, and also what should the dentist do while the assistant is busy? How can all four hands be most effectively used in order to shorten the total working time? Remember that the best teamwork will frequently involve the dentist helping—doing things for the dental assistant; not just the assistant helping the doctor. If either member of the team comes to a point where he (or she) has nothing to do momentarily, and the other member is busy, the first one should try to do something that will speed things up later on. For example, if the doctor is contouring a matrix band, and everything else is ready, the assistant could remove the used burs from the handpiece in anticipation of cleaning up for the next patient or even another type of bur or stone for this patient. If all else is done, and the DA is busy preparing something, say, mixing a cement base, the dentist might remove the bur, etc. Try to plan ahead and work together in this manner for real speed and competency.

If you and the doctor will take the time to go through each

separate procedure this way on paper, you will find yourselves much faster and better at the chair. True, you may find things do not quite work out exactly at the chair as you had planned, but it will usually require very little alteration to make things better. After doing this only a very few times, you both will become so automatic in your planning and thinking ahead that it will be second nature and your total efficiency will multiply rapidly.

Operatory Arrangements

In order to be most effective with your doctor, you must actually be able to be practically as close to the patient as he is, and be able to see most everything the doctor does. In this way you can see what phase or task he is performing and be in a much better position (relatively, as well as figuratively) to anticipate him and help him.

In other words, if there is a cuspidor between you and the patient and the dentist, you may likely either end the day with a very sore back and aching arms, or else you will not have assisted him as much as would be desired. You must do whatever is possible and practical to get you closer and more convenient to the operating scene. Let's talk about a few of the ways you can do this.

The ideal: your dentist buys a new contour-type chair, console, stools (two, not one, so you have one too), instrument trays and adequate counter top space. All of these are conveniently arranged around the treatment room so that the patient's head is the center focus. Then the dentist is on one side with the patient's head more or less cradled in his lap (on the chair's head rest naturally) and you are on the opposite side in about a three o'clock position. If you two can see fit to do so, you both should be positioned so that your legs more or less intertwine. You should be that close! Thank heavens for pantsuits!

Now, position either a cervical tray or a mobile stand of some sort just at your lap if you're at the three o'clock position, or at your right wrist if you're at two o'clock. This is considering the dentist works right handed, of course. The point is, the tray of hand instruments must be as close to you as convenient so you can merely drop your fingers and you'll have an instrument. You do not want to move your arm or hand more than six inches to get an instrument.

The handpieces and suction apparatus should be readily available to you with your left hand so you can hand the doctor these as need be. In this manner you will need to do very little movement for the primary instrumentation. If you need to have additional instruments, they are in a cabinet drawer no further than a three-quarter arm's length reach. This is made possible by either a mobile cabinet or close proximity of the dental drawers.

Arrange the drawers so the most frequently used pieces of equipment are most convenient and readily accessible. You do not want to have to go digging down into the back for, say, a special retainer, or a new matrix band.

Finally, if you have all of this, make sure it is all mobile enough so that you can easily get up and leave and return if you need to. If the dentist needs some piece of equipment not immediately present, and it takes you two minutes to push and lay everything aside, get it and return to your starting position, you've lost the game. The room must be large enough to permit you free and easy movement.

If your doctor buys a unit console of the type that has the handpieces and evacuation equipment at the rear of the chair, you will possibly need a convenient tray that will move more freely than a mobile cabinet. In such a situation make certain your stool is an easily rotating one, so you can swivel on it easily and still keep all your hand instruments within an easy grasp.

If your doctor has gone to the expense of investing in all of the above equipment in at least two of his operatories, you are certainly sitting pretty. Your employer is to be complemented for his foresight. You are working in the ideal situation.

Unfortunately, however, such an outlay is quite costly and it may be your office has only one such room, or perhaps none at all. Your task therefore becomes to do what you can to convert what you have to increase its efficiency and still spend a bare minimum of the doctor's dollars. Here are a few suggestions. You can put many of these into practice with no major cost, and some will require some expense, but you should think out each one carefully before offering it to your employer. Whatever you do will have a direct effect on him—pro or con—and you must be sure to have his approval—even it it's only "we'll try it a time or two" type of go-ahead.

The first consideration is your access to the patient and the operating field. This must be if you are to be effective, whether you and the doctor stand or sit.

The most frequently occurring obstacle is the cuspidor on the old upright unit. This will move somewhat out of your way, but invariably you must pull back out of the way in order for the patient to empty his mouth.

If you are sitting down at the chair, it becomes quickly apparent that this becomes an almost unbelievable problem. You have a lap full of instruments plus water or air syringe plus perhaps holding the handpiece for the doctor and the patient needs to empty. Here you go, scrambling around hastily trying to move everything (including yourself) out of the way so you can swing the Big White Bowl around for the patient to use. Then back goes everything for a minute after which when you repeat the whole mess.

You should have a high-speed evacuator to be effective. These can be purchased for as little as $200 on a portable basis and are easily transportable from room to room. If your doctor will not buy one, then keep the Big White Bowl but adjust your total working manner so that it's readily available without your moving so much. You'll have to sit or stand at a more or less one o'clock position and probably have to lean over toward the patient, but you will at least be able to let the patient spit with a minimum of trouble.

If you can finagle an evacuator, then you should get the BWB taken off. It's easy to do, and your local supply house would probably do it for you. Here's how it is done: first turn the water off! Take off the Bowl and place it in your farthest corner of a dark closet. Cover it with boxes so you will forget where it is. Have the repair man cap the water pipe and double check for leakage. The drain need not be closed. Your unit will be left with a gaping hole in its side, so have a local tinsmith (or an air conditioning or heating man) make you a tin cover to slip into the hole. He can design the edges so that the part will snap securely into place and stay there, yet not damage the unit. Then get the proper color of paint from the supply house and paint it (two or three coats), and you will have a nice enough looking corner and no BWB!

Actually, do not forget entirely where the BWB is stored, and don't throw it away, because someday your doctor may want to sell the unit *in toto* and you can reinstall The Bowl.

You might run into a slight problem with a few of the doctor's patients when they have a desire to spit and can't find the BWB. After they overcome their look of terror, ask them to lean back and you'll clean their mouth for them with you high speed suction tip. (The Pelton & Crane "Tip-a-dillo" is helpful too.) If you wish to provide one, you can get a "vac-u-cup" that is simply a funnel that attaches to the evacuator pipe. The patients then can have their own individual BWB. Please be sure to buy the funnel-shaped Lily cups that go with it so it will remain sanitary. These special cups, incidentally, have a hole in the bottom so the "stuff" goes down the drain.

Other "personal cuspidors" have water tips added for a more realistic effect, and can be somewhat quieter but are really no more effective.

I will point out that a rather disconcerting sound is effected with the vacuum cup on the high-speed evacuator, but the advantage of the patient's being able to use it while prone outweighs the problem.

Okay, you've got this BWB detail eliminated, but you still have the bracket arm and table frequently in the way. This is especially so if your doctor has the patient lying back. You can tilt the chair back far enough to raise the patient's legs into the table or bracket arm. Have the table removed in a similar fashion as the BWB. Be sure to have the gas shut off to the burner if there is one on the bracket arm. Also, of course, any electrical or water or air sources should be shut off. Then you'll have a rather streamlined upright unit that interferes with you only slightly.

This unit alteration may not be possible with every type of unit, but will certainly cover the vast majority.

It has been proven quite beneficial to all concerned if the patient can be in a supine position (or at least nearly so) when being treated. He is more relaxed, easier to work on, and is frankly less likely to suffer ill effects from the treatment or injections. But the old-type standard dental chair doesn't really offer much comfort in this position, so it is helpful to try to get your doctor to convert it to a more comfortable lounge type.

This doesn't require an enormous expenditure for a new top or base or even a new chair altogether. Check with a couple of supply houses or even in your doctor's journals and you'll find a number of seat backs that are easily adaptable to the standard chair. Then you can simply push the back rest lever to lower the back instead of relying on an electric switch. It's not as easy, but considerably cheaper.

When you do stretch the patient back like this, however, you'll more than likely find him complaining of having his stomach or thigh muscles stretched. It becomes obvious very quickly that you also need to stretch out the legs of your patient. Here again, you can buy economical supports to simply drop onto the foot rest of the chair and it will automatically become a lounge chair. Incidentally, if needed, it only takes five seconds to remove this leg support and return to an upright-type chair if you wish to do so.

Total expense for back and leg support can be less than $300, and except for the lack of motorized movement, will be as effective as the more costly modern lounge-type chairs.

Okay, you have connected the unit, and the chair, and you now have access to the patient, but you still need your instruments accessible to you. Here's what to do:

For a small cost you can purchase a tray and an extension arm. This is made by several different companies, and is quite handy. You simply screw its base into the wall at a predetermined level above the floor. (You need to carefully decide at exactly what level you want it, because you will not be able to easily change it without possibly messing up the plaster or wall board.) Then you place your instruments (or instrument trays) on this main tray and move it out from the wall in any direction over a full span of 180 degrees. It will normally extend about three and one-half feet, but additional extension arms can be added if need be. Try not to add extra extensions though, because it will pick up additional instability simply due to its longer length. It may have a tendency to "bounce" if you drop something on it.

Many offices use two or even three such extending trays—one

for the doctor's side if he desires, and one or even two for the assistant.

If possible, a mobile cabinet is helpful. It will carry the most widely used supplies: amalgam, silicates, cements, wedges, etc. If this is not a possibility, try to get a carpenter to construct a couple or three small compartmented boxes for you. These can be of a size to fit onto the tops of the tray as an extension arm, and deep enough to hold, say, a bottle of cement, and with enough compartments to keep many separate items. Then if your doctor is doing silicates, for instance, you can get out the instruments you expect him to use and place these on the tray nearest the patient's head, and get out your silicate supply box and place it on the other tray near your right side. Everything will be very handy to you, yet freely movable in case you need to leave quickly.

In order to have adequate counter space, it is simple and quite economical to have a large 4 x 8 piece of plywood, 3/4 inch thick cut down to the size and shape you desire and then mounted with sturdy wall brackets and covered with Formica. If your doctor already has a floor cabinet there, you can add this counter top around it so efficiently that it appears to be almost built in. Many offices have this made into an L-shape, so that the doctor has some space, but the assistant's side can be almost the full length of the room.

This counter would be built at any level you or your doctor desired, but remember to double check that the extension trays will fold up under it without bumping.

What I have tried to put across to you here is that if you feel that for whatever reasons your dentist will not or cannot go to the heavy expense of modern equipment needed for the most efficient dental production, it is possible to create a near similarity quite cheaply. You can at least point out some of the above information to him. In this way you may get started on the road to greater efficiency and production. Also in the manner described above he can do it on a piecemeal basis—a little at a time. He can try the back rest, or the leg support, then add the high-speed evacuator, then maybe the vac-u-cup, and so on, feeling his way along. If he becomes doubtful along the way, very little expense has been made.

Incidentally, although very fine dental stools can be purchased at a cost of $300-$400, quite adequate ones can be obtained for less than $50-$60 at your local office equipment house. Those are really secretarial or typist chairs, and perhaps do not work as smoothly or have as much chrome, but usually are nearly as comfortable, and can provide very adequate seating.

Typical Tray Setups You Can Use

As you and your dentist begin to develop your streamlined and effective procedures, you should also look into the possibilities of working directly from prearranged tray setups. For such setups you should first decide exactly which instruments are most commonly used by your doctor, and then decide which ones are only rarely used or needed. The main thing you need to note is that to have an excessive number of instruments on each tray can actually be rather inefficient in the long run. For instance, if you are continually having to wash and sterilize only six instruments that you use only once every two weeks, yet are on each and every tray, you can rather quickly chalk up a lot of wasted time and motion. It would be better to place on the normal trays only the most important, key instruments that you can reasonably expect to use eighty-five to ninety percent of the time. Then have the additional tools and instruments readily available at arms' length in a nearby cabinet or drawer. If you need the additional spoon or chisel, you need it right now, not after you dig through four drawers hunting for it.

If you have difficulty in deciding which are the key instruments, ask your dentist—after you have explained your purpose.

The following section contains some examples of typical tray setups for a dental office. You probably will not wish to copy these exactly, because of the fact that each dentist may wish to adapt his hands to other tools or techniques. The main purpose here is to give you a starting point. As you will note as you scan through these photographs, no specific instruments are named, but rather generalities are used, for easy adaptation by you and your office.

Prophylaxis tray (Figure 11-2). From left to right, mouth

mirror, explorer, pick-ups (cotton pliers), two different scalers, dappen dish for pumice (pumice on one side, polishing chalk later on the other side)—the sticky pumice will not fall out, and you can save having to wash and sterilize two instruments or dishes here). A couple of sponges for wiping instruments, a polishing angle and new cup, and lastly a saliva ejector.

Amalgams (Figure 11-3). Left to right—two mouth mirrors (one for the doctor, and one for the assistant, retraction, etc.), pick-ups, explorer, spoon excavator. Above these are a dappen dish (flat) containing commonly used burs for this procedure, and a bur changer. The dish is flat for easy access to the burs. This completes all of the cavity preparation instruments. The remaining instruments on the tray are directed toward filling and completing the restoration. The preparation instruments are not likely to be used again and can be removed from the tray or at least moved to a spot on the tray where they will not be in the way. Now you see the matrix retainers and bands and wedges most frequently needed, followed by pluggers, and amalgam carver. The pliers are used for placing the wedges as well as removing them and the matrix bands, and could have been placed between the retainers and the pluggers just as well. The Kelly forceps contain a "glob" of cotton to be used to smooth down the carving. There follows a high-speed evacuation tip plus a saliva ejector. The final instrument is a periodontal probe which can be used for placing CaOH or ZOE liners under fillings. It could be placed between the matrix retainers and the pluggers also, but is most frequently picked up initially by the dental assistant, and is therefore located immediately adjacent to her relative position at the chair.

Amalgams, Silicates, Cementing Combinations (Figure 11-4). For the patient where your dentist will be placing amalgams, and silicates (or composites or resins) as well as seating and cementing castings all in the same appointment, one tray is quite adequate, and two or three separate trays become an unnecessary burden and waste. Two mirrors, explorer, pick-ups, spoon excavator, amalgam pluggers, and carver. Trimming chisel. Flat dappen dish and anticipated burs and bur changer. Grinding stones for adjusting the castings. Optional cotton rolls. Articulating paper. Matrix bands and retainers, and plastic instrument. Temporary crown or cement removing instrument. High-speed evacuator tip, and saliva ejector and finally a liner applicator, and dental floss.

Silicates, Resins, Composits (Figure 11-5). Two mouth mirrors, explorer, pick-ups, spoon excavator. Optional cotton rolls, flat dappen dish with bur changer and anticipated burs and trimming stone. Celluloid strip and strip holder if desired. Plastic instrument and trimming chisel, followed by the suction tip, saliva ejector and liner applicator.

Preparations and Impressions (Figure 11-6). Two mirrors, explorer, pick-ups, spoon excavator. Next an injection syringe for the impression material, and an impression tray. Dappen dish, bur changer and burs, and cotton rolls. Contouring pliers for the temporary aluminum crown, suction tip, saliva ejector, and liner applicator.

Cementation (Figure 11-7). Two mouth mirrors, explorer, pick-ups temporary crown or cement remover, spoon. Cotton rolls, gold-trimming burs, reducing stones. Next, dental floss, articulating paper and rubber wheel for biting pressure at cementation. Next come crown-removing pliers that could just as easily be placed beside the cement remover on the tray. Then follow the saliva ejector and liner applicator.

Periodontal Flap Surgery (Figure 11-8). A mouth mirror and pick-ups, followed by a scalpel with the appropriate blade as determined by the dentist. Periosteal elevator, large curette, and a small curette. Bone bur, and then needle holder, surgical scissors, suture, sponges and a small-tipped high-speed evacuator tip.

Endodontia (Figure 11-9). First the rubber dam punch and rubber dam would be used, followed by the appropriate rubber dam clamp, clamp forcep, and frame. Next cotton swabs for sterilizing the rubber dam, and the saliva ejector for the patient's mouth. Now, mouth mirror, explorer, and a long-shafted spoon and the flat dappen dish and burs for removing temporary filling or pulpal tissue and such. Splinter forceps for grasping root canal instruments, points, etc. Appropriate paper points, trial filling points, irrigating syringes and X-ray film complete the basic tray setup.

Mandibular First or Second Molar Extraction (Figure 11-10).

Mirror, pick-ups, tissue-retraction elevator, tooth elevator, forceps, curette, sponges, and evacuator.

Maxillary Molar Extraction (Figure 11-11). Mirror, pick-ups, periosteal elevator, tooth elevator, forceps, curette, sponges and evacuator tip are usually all that are needed here.

Maxillary Anterior or Cuspid Extraction (Figure 11-12). The only change here over that of the maxillary molar or premolar tray is the switch to a different forcep.

Mandibular Anterior or Cuspid Extraction (Figure 11-13). This tray setup is identical to that of the maxillary anterior or cuspid tray except for the forcep.

Maxillary Bicuspid, Cuspid, Anterior Extraction (Figure 11-14). The purpose of this photograph which is identical to those of the mandibular and maxillary anterior or cuspid extraction trays is to point out that trays can be built around individual forceps, rather than around the specific tooth to be removed. If your doctor has a bare minimum number of forceps and must make certain ones do for multiple teeth, then you can simply set up a tray with whatever forceps he has available that can be used and that will suffice.

Preliminary (Snap) Impressions (Figure 11-15). You will usually be able to set up a tray such as this by beginning with medium-sized impression trays (universal). There will naturally be occasions when your doctor will call for a larger or smaller size, but most will fit this medium size. Two separate rubber bowls and two mixing spatulas will save you some messy cleanup, and time, in the operatory while the patient is there watching. After all, alginate is pretty messy stuff. Many offices buy alginate in bulk cans and measure out various scoops whenever an impression is to be taken. This can use up a considerable amount of time while the dentist is waiting, and it frequently costs more money to use the prepackaged types, so it will likely pay you to buy some small paper bags and place in each one premeasured amounts of alginate from the bulk canisters. These paper bags are quite cheap and can be used over and over again. If you have concern about shelf life of the material in the bags after removing them from the bulk can, then find an old alginate (or other) can that has been emptied, and place the bags with alginate inside this can and close the lid. This will provide you with as much shelf life as the original bulk can, as long as you handle all the bags and alginate with dry hands.

Don't forget the water measuring cup on the tray.

Final Impressions for Complete Dentures (Figure 11-16). Mouth mirror, ample stick compound, laboratory knife, impression cream, paper mixing pad, tongue blade mixing spatulas, rubber bowl (if your dentist prefers to have you wrap the impressions in a wet paper towel after taking them—it helps keep the trays from getting "scattered" over the entire counter this way), and Vaseline or lubricant for the patient's face and lips, and the dentist's and your hands. Naturally, if your dentist prefers other types of final impressions, your tray should contain the proper materials accordingly.

Your own imagination in your office can help you to set up trays best. You will no doubt want to have several duplicates of the most frequently used types. If you run out of, say, amalgam trays some afternoon and do not have time to go to the sterilizing center to sterilize the instruments for one of the used trays, you can pull a combination tray, such as "amalgam, silicate, cement" tray. While this will necessitate sterilizing unused instruments later, the key to real production is to have the team operating effectively while the patient is there, so this is better.

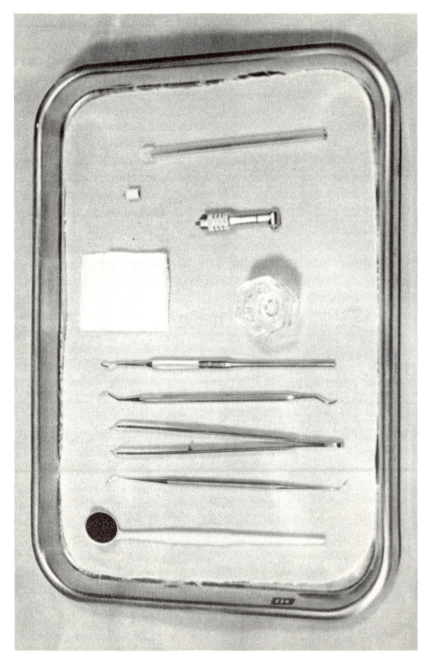

Figure 11-2:   Prophylaxis

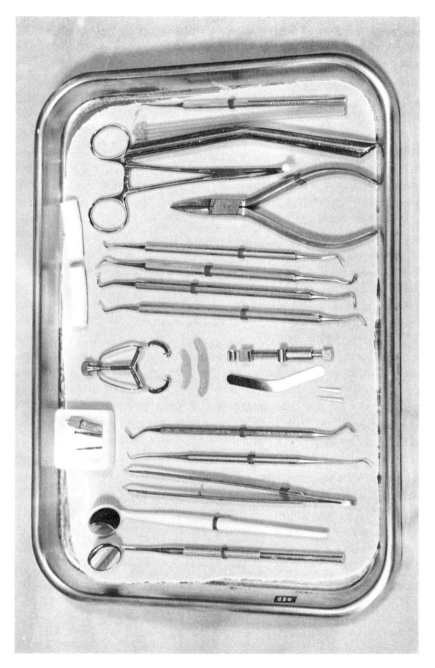

Figure 11-3:   Amalgams

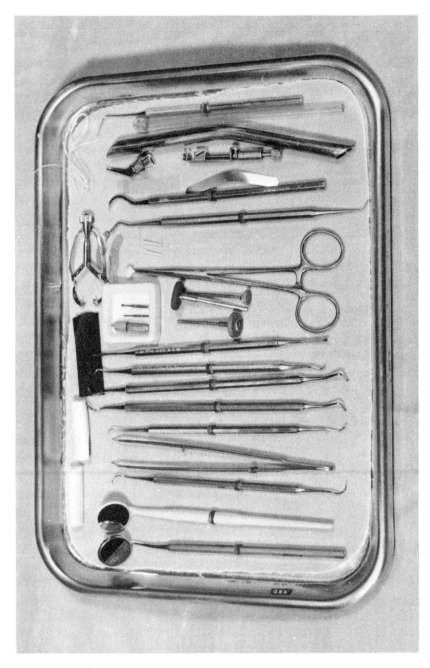

Figure 11-4:   Amalgams, Silicates, and Cementing

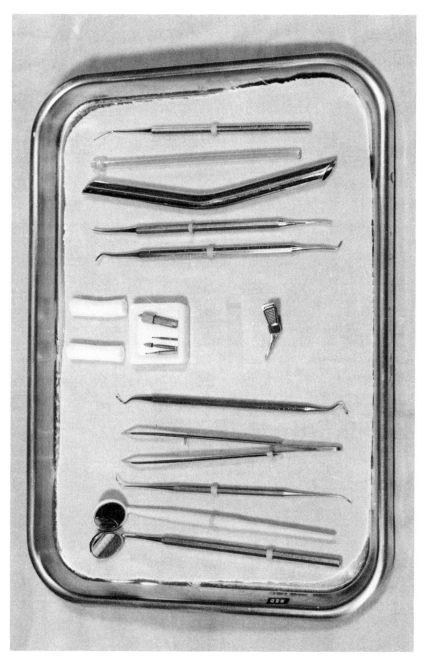

Figure 11-5:   Silicates, Plastics, and Composits

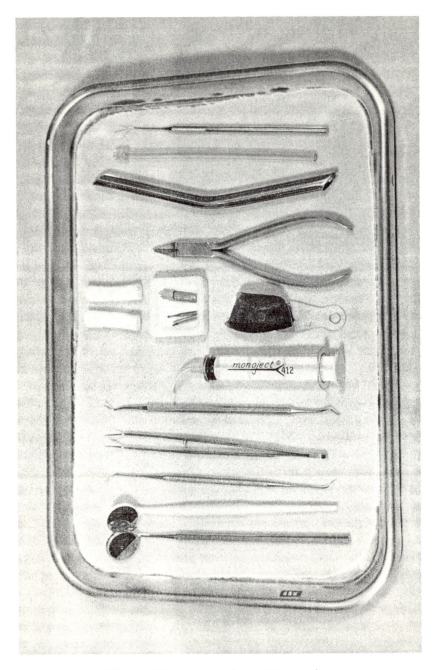

Figure 11-6:   Preparation and Impression

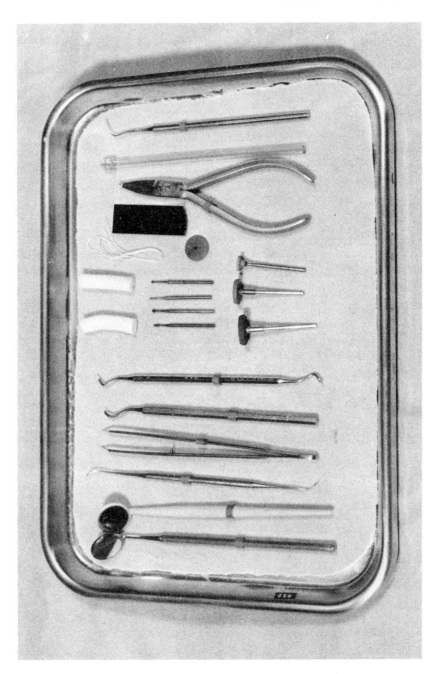

Figure 11-7:   Cementation

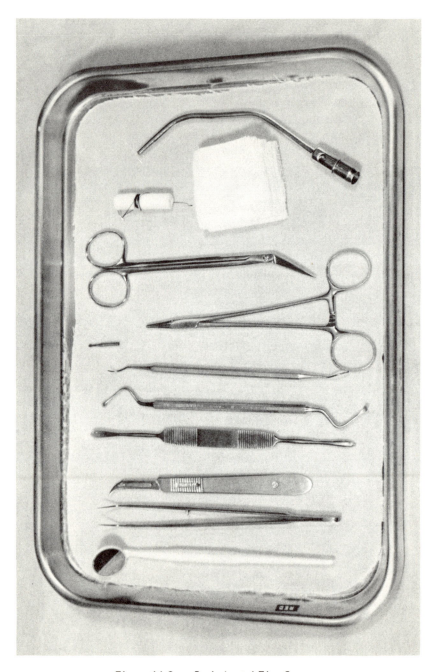

Figure 11-8:   Periodontal Flap Surgery

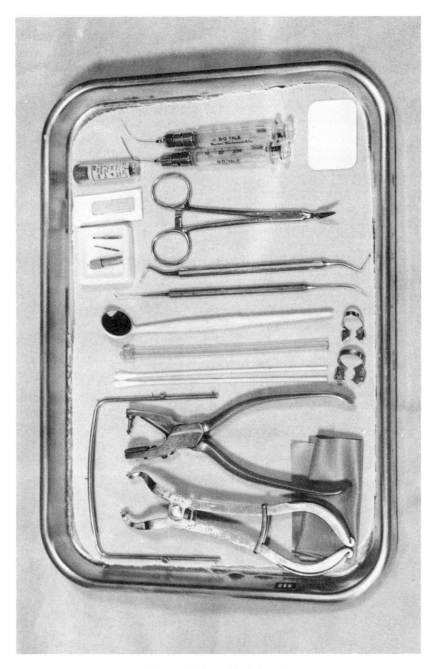

Figure 11-9: Endodontia

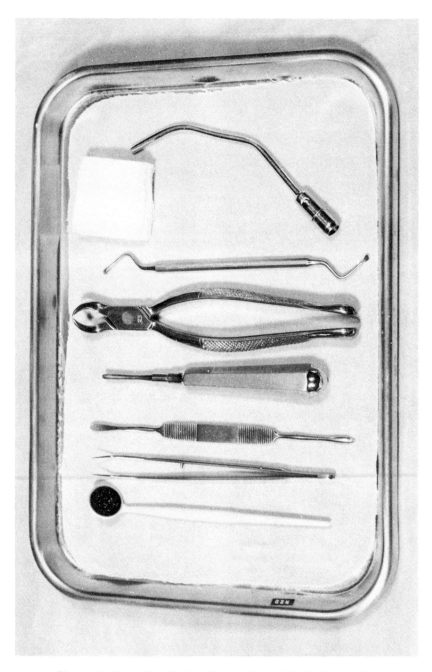

Figure 11-10:   Mandibular First or Second Molar Extraction

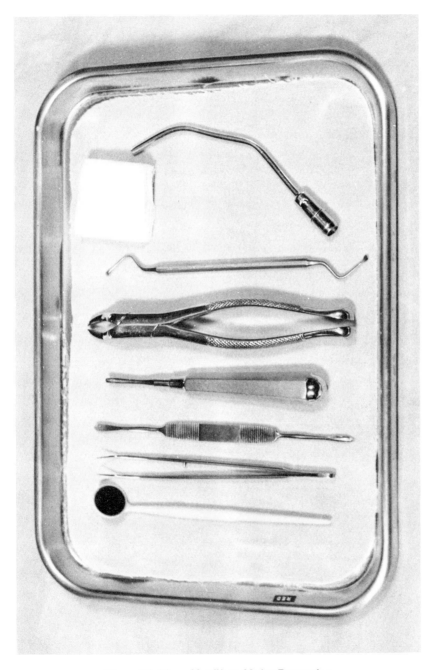

Figure 11-11: Maxillary Molar Extraction

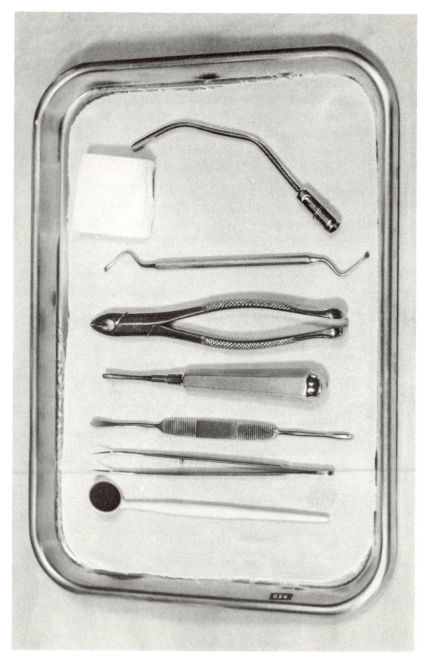

Figure 11-12:   Maxillary Anterior or Cuspid Extraction

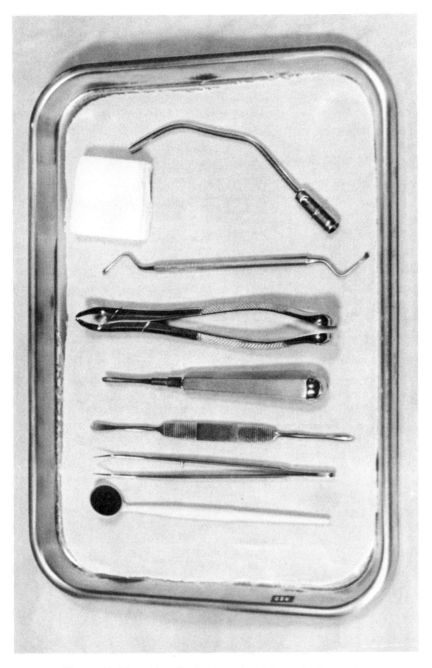

Figure 11-13: Mandibular Anterior, Biscuspid Extraction

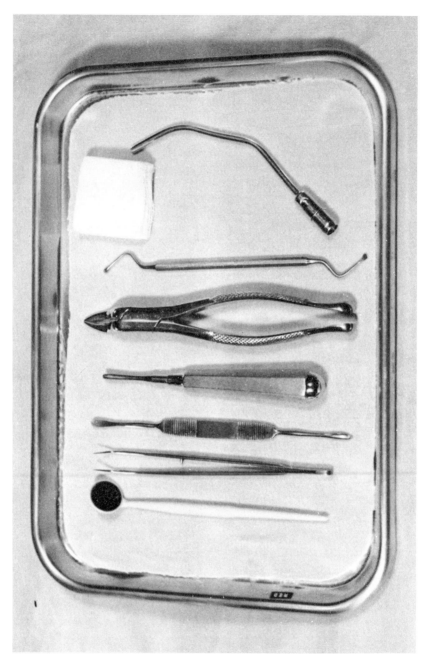

Figure 11-14: Maxillary Bicuspid, Cuspid, Anterior Extraction

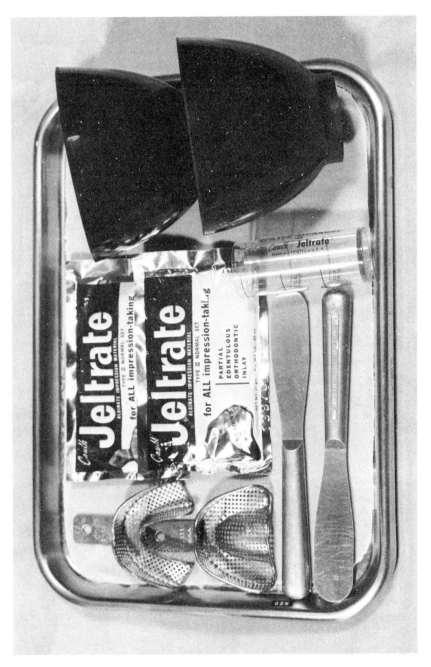

Figure 11-15: Snap or Preliminary Impressions

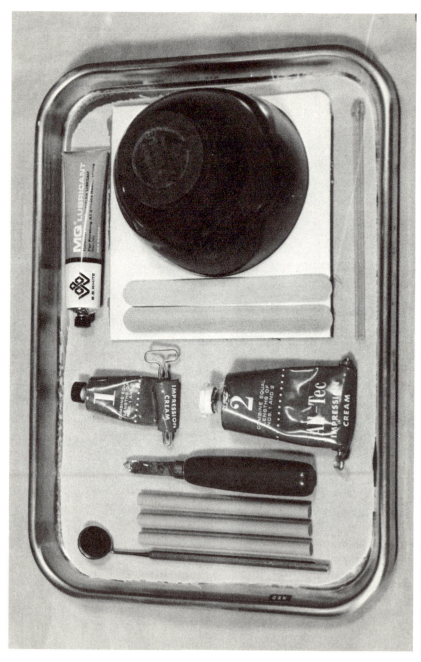

Figure 11-16:   Final Impressions for Complete Dentures

12 | *The Four-Handed Technique*

Its Purpose

With the advent of the high-speed handpiece, and a few pioneer studies about time and motion in the dental office, certain radical changes began to take place. These basically had their beginnings in the middle 1950s and have evolved rapidly in the 1960s to now. Dentistry as a profession has come to realize that it can no longer function adequately with the one-chair, one-man office. With the almost overwhelming mass of patients needing dentistry across the country, a dentist truly has a moral and ethical obligation to work faster (more efficiently, with quality as good as ever) and to treat more patients each week or month. In other words, each dentist should produce his absolute maximum at all times.

The realization has come, however, that no one man can produce consistently at such a pace without adequate help. If his load is heavy, and he tries to do all the chores, he will soon either let his work become slipshod or else run the risk of physical and possibly emotional and mental breakdown. So, fortunately, the profession has had enough foresight to bring the dental assistant more obviously into the picture.

You DAs are no longer expected to just be "the girl," and follow the doctor around and clean up afterward. You have become true assistants in every sense of the word. This is where the expression "four-handed dentistry" comes in.

Now, in today's up-to-date dental offices, the DA is really two extra hands of the dentist. In many offices, a second chairside DA or "rover" becomes the fifth and sixth hands. In this manner all effort is made to permit the dentist to function at his utmost efficiency, with absolutely minimized lost motion, yet have his labors made as easy as possible on him physically and mentally. This is not to say he is lazy (yours may be), but that it behooves you to keep your employer healthy for the longest number of years possible and in an active practice. If he has his work made easier for him, he is more likely to live longer. This favors his family, you, as well as the patients who need him. The technique of four-handed dentistry can help everyone.

Its Pitfalls

The real key to the four-handed technique is that same old cliché, "teamwork." As you become two more of the dentist's hands, you must also become an outgrowth of his mind. You must convince him that he must give some thought to your mind also. You must help each other in order to accomplish the best results.

So discuss the various details of your duties (yours and his) from time to time and try to smooth out rough areas of procedures. If some particular instrument transfer seems awkward to you, then the two of you should discuss it and perhaps develop an alternate transfer that will work more smoothly. If he consistently creates a particular situation that causes you a lot of delay or unnecessary (in your eyes) work, see if the two of you can even this out. Never forget that he is your employer, and handle it quite tactfully, but he should be made to realize that if you waste time, it is actually his time (and money) he is losing.

A very important point for you to know, therefore, is to keep a clear and alert mind about every movement you and the doctor make during your four-handed procedures and try to improve each one. Keep asking yourself: "Why am I doing this? How could it be done differently? Would it be better another way?" Also ask yourself, "If the doctor did such and such, would I be able to help him better?"

A critical pitfall in four-handed is the fact that the DA just might not apply herself to her tasks. She might be contented to sit back and let the dentist direct traffic and all of the movements around the patient. She might have no initiative whatsoever. Frankly, whether the doctor realizes it or not, he just might be better off with someone else.

Another problem you frequently see is that four hands in one mouth has a tendency to get a little crowded. There are times when you simply must give a little and let the doctor do it by himself. Don't be "put out" or chagrined if he moves you out of the mouth momentarily. It's probably just that he needs a little more room to work. Certainly you want to do your job of, say, suctioning and retracting as inconspicuously as possible. For instance, if you can combine retractions with the suction tip and maintain the vacuum plus safety, that's all to the better, but make sure you are at the maximum effectiveness on both counts.

If your dentist has always practiced stand-up two-handed dentistry, you may find it impossible for him to alter his technique. It can be done certainly, but it is difficult to change a method of operating followed for many years. You might make attempts to switch him over, as it will certainly make your own work easier, but if he feels he just doesn't want to change, then so be it. Remember, good or bad, it is his life and his practice. You must do everything possible to help him and to make his job easier. But you cannot make him alter his procedures if he doesn't want to. You might keep trying, however, with gentle hints and nudges ever so often. Maybe he'll come around after all.

How You Can Better the Examination

One of the keys to the successful completion of a case by the dentist is a successful beginning. This means that if the patient is started properly, he will more likely appreciate the efforts of the dentist and have confidence in him and follow through with the acceptance of his recommendations. Your direct involvement in the mouth examination can help immensely.

As you are no doubt aware, the doctor needs to dry each

tooth prior to his examination of it. This does several things: it blows away the saliva so the fissures of the tooth can be inspected. It will turn decalcified tooth (predecay) chalky, and make it more obvious. It makes it possible to see the plaque that is there. If there are any cracks in the enamel, they can be seen more easily when dry. The blast of air can indicate a tooth that is cold-sensitive (and how!) and the blast of air can also show the integrity of the gingival margin.

Your job: dry each tooth for the doctor. He can then hold the mouth mirror and explorer and examine each tooth more rapidly and efficiently than if he had to lay the explorer down, pick up the air syringe, dry the tooth, then go back to the explorer. You can simplify the exam even more if you place cotton rolls in appropriate salivary ducts prior to the drying. This way your doctor can frequently cover an entire quadrant or even arch with very little wasted motion. Don't forget though what you're trying to do: you are drying the tooth completely for the doctor. Please do not miss some areas—be thorough.

Step number two is to record his findings. Have your charts and pencils and pens readily available and set to go. He will most likely always start in the same area, say, maxillary right third molar, and work his way around the upper arch completely before moving to the lower arch.

You should speak to him first about this, but a good suggestion would be to utilize the "dictated" exam. This way he moves from tooth to tooth and calls out to you *everything* he sees. He can record it on a dictaphone or tape recorder for later transfer to charts, but you can easily record it as he progresses.

You will need a specially prepared paper for your recordings. You can do it in block form, with thirty-two blocks on the sheet, or you can simply have each tooth number or label on a separate line. You record all his pertinent findings either in longhand, or in symbols or code.

The doctor's exam will then go something like this:

Maxillary right third molar—missing

Maxillary right second molar—disto-occlusal caries; mesio-occlusal amalgam—worn, chipped margins

Maxillary right first molar—large MOD amalgam; thin mesiobuccal cusp.

Tooth number 4, MOD inlay, cervical erosion, needs restoration

Number 5, MO amalgam, darkened enamel on facial; should have crown

Number 6, appears okay

Number 7, distal filling, mesial caries

Number 8, darkened due to endodontia, large MIL plastic worn and discolored; severe mottling at labial gum line; should have post-crown

and so on

Now what has been accomplished is this: you have recorded basically everything describable about each tooth. This will greatly aid the doctor when he is reading the films and preparing the case for his presentation. In addition to recording existing work and decay, you have noted out of the ordinary things that cannot be easily symbolized on a dental chart. Such notations will help the dentist to recall each specific tooth far better than a simple X-ray film and symbolized dental chart.

One other aspect—and a very important one—is that you, and he (the patient) hears it in a third-party situation. The doctor is describing to you specific points about each tooth and not trying to impress the patient. In reality, of course, the patient is being subtly prepared for the case presentation at this particular time. For instance, if the doctor says, "Number 14 should have a casting for reinforcement of that lingual cusp," and says it to you, and not to the patient, you can bet your bottom dollar the patient will be quite interested at presentation when he speaks of castings, inlays, crowns and the like.

In other words, it is like sowing little seeds of curiosity that will blossom into conscientious concern and interest at presentation. The doctor is much more likely to convince the patient on the idea of complete rehabilitation dentistry this way.

Another example would be when Mrs. Jones needs a fixed bridge on the lower left. Your doctor might describe it as follows: "Number 18 has a large amalgam covering the mesial and the distal as well as the occlusal surfaces [you record on MOD amalgam]. The molar beside it is missing [#19—missing] and it has shifted its normal position in the mouth and has tilted forward. The opposing tooth [#14] has begun to sag [patient's eyes open slightly wider] and a bridge needs to be built. [Place appropriate brackets.] It would attach to the bicuspid which has a disto-occlusal amalgam that is leaking. [Indicate #20 with a defective DO amalgam.] Since it comes so close to the front of the mouth [he may even say "close to the smile"] a porcelain bridge would probably be better than a gold one."

Now this patient has become aware of the fact that she has numerous areas of her teeth already filled, her mouth is changing shape, and there is something known as a bridge that can be made of gold or porcelain. She'll go straight home and look at her mouth in a mirror. When the dentist sees her next and discusses a fixed bridge, she'll be very attentive.

Likewise, the third-party description is effective for patients with periodontal disease as the doctor describes "deep pockets" (record millimeter depth) or loose teeth (record mobility).

If you arrange it with your doctor, the effectiveness of the examination can be increased by reversing the situation. This time you ask the doctor pertinent questions, "Doctor, are there any weak cusps?" "Are there any loose teeth?" "Should any teeth have castings?" "Has that missing tooth caused any problems?"

When he answers these leading questions (remember, the two of you are more or less talking over the patient's head, but not specifically *to* him) you just know the patient's curiosity will be aroused.

To really impress the patient on the thoroughness of your office, you should also ask specific questions about extra-dental things. "Doctor, do you see any lesions in the mouth?" "Is there any abnormality present?" "What is the condition of the soft tissue?" "Saliva?" "Occlusion?" "Assymmetry?" "Diastemata?" "Overlapping teeth?" "Any sign of cancer?" "Any sign of physical diseases present?"

In this way the patient *knows* your dentist is absolutely thorough. You and I know that these things are normally looked for anyway, but nothing is usually said to the patient unless there is a specific problem noted. Now she knows (and appreciates) that all of his diagnostic skills are being put to use. She truly knows she has had an absolutely top-drawer examination (and is most frequently quite willing to pay the fee for it).

To aid you as well as the doctor in this line, you should type up a checklist for everything your doctor wants to include in his standard examination. Then, you can simply go down the list, item by item, and be confident that the patient referred by Mrs. Jones received every bit as thorough an exam as she did.

Be certain you and your doctor have discussed the questions completely. You must never ask a question (such as some of the above) after he has apparently finished his examination. This might have a tendency to make him appear to have forgotten something and that you had to remind him. Frankly that might make him forget to let you keep your job!

13

Guidelines for Equipment Care

The Case for Care Versus Neglect

In the everyday hustle and bustle of the average dental office, your dentist (and you too, certainly) is constantly being hammered with pressures. His day is tension, tension, tension. His work is tedious and usually difficult—particularly if he is trying to do his best. Therefore he is usually looking for ways to make his day just a little bit easier and smoother. Likewise you should try to smooth it out, and help to prevent or eliminate all possible and potential frustrations.

And nothing can be quite so frustrating and tension-producing as equipment malfunction right smack in the middle of a serious procedure. In addition, it can be a source of embarrassment for him if his equipment runs down from apparent lack of care.

Therefore it becomes your solemn duty to maintain every item of equipment in the entire office working and in tip-top condition at all times. If any problem develops due to poor maintenance, you must consider it your fault. Please don't do such a thing to your doctor. Take proper care of his equipment.

Practically every piece of equipment purchased by the dentist will be accompanied by literature about its care. This information is included because most equipment manufacturers have studied the situation carefully and know exactly what type care and upkeep are required to keep it in first-class working order. In addition, most equipment is under a warranty and you must observe prescribed care rules in order to keep the warranty in effect.

Time after time it has been shown that equipment manufactured today will normally serve faithfully for years and years, patient after patient if it is only cared for as it was designed to be.

Another point in favor of proper care is the enormous expenditure required for equipment purchase. It is sheer waste to neglect a fine machine of any type or description.

Many people feel that simple neglect is the thing that will cause equipment failure. Naturally this is an important concern, but another problem is the wrong kind of treatment. If a piece of machinery is pushed beyond its design limits too often, it will break down. Never use a tool for something other than for what it was designed. For example, a screwdriver is not to be used as an enamel chisel and an enamel chisel is not to be used as a screwdriver—even though it is just the right size for that tiny screw. Screwdrivers are cheap—chisels are expensive.

How to Utilize Cleaners

Cleanliness is next to Godliness and isn't your dental office heavenly? You have certainly been well-coached in keeping instruments clean and sterile and dust-free, and the floors and furniture clean, but you must also take care to keep the mechanisms of the office clean. This refers to any moving part of any piece of equipment regardless of size or shape or usage.

It is totally impossible to keep dust particles out of the office. And it is also complicating to find tooth dust debris in a handpiece. This hard enamel dust can certainly create wear and tear on a geared mechanism quickly. Therefore, one major chore to be done is to clean the handpieces daily. This especially applies to the slower speed, heavy-torque types. The more modern air turbines are relatively self-cleaning and lubricating, but you must do some special turbine cleaning with some of the earlier models. Check the literature that came with each specific handpiece if it is available; otherwise ask your dealer for instructions. If he cannot help you, write to the manufacturer.

There are special handpiece cleaners available, and you should stick with them. Don't try to substitute cheaper cleaners, because special metal alloys are used and might be harmed by some wrong solution.

If you will look closely at the handpieces, you will find small openings built in for lubrication. These are also used for the insertion of cleaner. The key is to wash out all of the old oil, junk, and debris, and then let as much as possible of the nonlubricating cleanser drain off before replacing the oil. If a pore is clogged, a small wire or smooth broach will help to free it. If the cleaner misses reaching any part of the handpiece, it won't be cleaned, will it?

About once a month (you should follow a definite planned schedule) you should break the handpieces down. This means to take them apart as much as is practical, and thoroughly inspect and hand clean the working parts and gears. The daily treatment is mandatory, but will occasionally leave some small area of grime that just can't be removed without direct contact by hand. Clean each part until spotless and then wipe off all possible cleaner prior to reassembly. Incidentally, be certain you can (1) disassemble without bending or damaging any parts or sheaths, and (2) reassemble. A clean handpiece in ten pieces on the work bench doesn't work too well. Here your doctor or the supply house representative can help you.

Note: Some manufacturers specifically prohibit disassembly of their handpieces. Follow the rules by all means—otherwise your doctor may lose the warranty (and the handpiece, if it becomes broken).

Most cleaners are not effective lubricants so whenever you run a handpiece in a jar of cleaner, do it slowly. Never operate a handpiece at high speed in cleaner, since once the lubricant and grime are flushed out, and only cleaner remains, you invite the tendency for the handpiece to wear inside on the bearings and gears.

If your office has belt-driven handpieces, remember that the belt pulleys receive enormous amounts of wear. They also pick up dust and lint which harm them. You should plan to keep these cleaned on a regular basis also. If you cannot take the separate pulleys off, then at least blow them forcefully with the compressed air syringe. Blow off all possible lint and grime, then use a small strip of cotton cloth (about 6″ x ¼″) that has been soaked in handpiece cleaner, and scrub over and around the pulley's shaft. Then drop two or three drops of cleaner onto the rotating axis and blast it again with the air syringe. Let it dry before re-oiling, and do not operate it without oiling.

How to Oil Properly

Oiling a piece of machinery or equipment can require a special knack. The fact is that too much oil can be almost as hazardous as too little. The key is just the right amount at just the right time.

After you have completed a thorough cleaning of the equipment or mechanical instrument, you will have two or more pieces of metal contacting each other. They rub and create (1) wear, (2) friction, and (3) heat. Oil will reduce the harm from all three to a minimum.

What you are striving for is not to have the pieces literally floating in lubricant, but a relatively thin layer of oil (or film) between parts. If you have sufficient film of the right consistency, it will remain on the metal for some time. This means that oil that is excessively thin will fly off or drip off very quickly and lose its effectiveness. Here's a point to remember: oil that is even partially mixed with leftover cleaner will become diluted and thinned and will not be as good as you need it to be. As I mentioned earlier, always let as much cleaner drip off or be wiped off as possible and practical prior to lubrication.

Oil has a tendency to gum up when it picks up floating dust particles and debris. When it does become gummy, it quickly increases the drag on the tool to force it to work harder and strain the motor or operator. In addition, it captures dirt particles and literally grinds them into the metal surfaces it is covering. This increased wear is naturally detrimental, so obviously you must keep oil changed frequently to prevent any gumming.

Don't forget this: if you have freshly cleaned and oiled a handpiece, please let it "drip dry" and then wipe it off thoroughly. All too frequently excess oil will remain on it and leave a pretty lousy taste for the patient. Heaven knows, they usually have a bad enough taste following treatment anyway. A suggestion here is to plan your work so that your cleaning and oiling are done immediately following the last patient at night. In the first place, you will be able to clean the handpiece easier since the junk on it will not have had an opportunity to dry out and harden as much, and secondly the excess oil will have an opportunity to drip off during the night. Just be certain to wipe it off carefully the next day prior to the doctor's first usage.

When you are oiling an instrument or piece of equipment always follow the specifications of the manufacturer. That is, use the proper thickness or viscosity of oil. Hopefully you or your doctor have preserved the original "specs" provided with the original purchase of the equipment. Contained within will be the correct type oil as recommended by the manufacturing firm. In many cases, the company will actually enclose an original starting amount of the specified lubricant. You simply need to reorder from time to time. Again, don't hesitate to consult your supply house for the lubricant or at least information about it. Otherwise you should write the specific manufacturing firm for their recommendation. This all may seem like a lot of trouble but it really is important if the doctor's equipment is to last as long as he hopes it will.

When speaking of lubrication we have a tendency to think primarily of the rapidly moving drills, motors, handpieces, etc., but there are many other areas of the office that need occasional oiling and greasing. These may be too numerous to describe here, but after a few suggestions, you should look around your office diligently and make a specific list. Then you can follow with your doctor's or the supply house's recommendation as to the frequency with which it should have some attention. This may be weekly, monthly, semiannually, or perhaps only annually.

Here are a few examples: the slides of the chair, the rotating points of the chair arms, the pedals on the floor rheostat, the finger activating levers on the water, and air syringe (internal pulleys or retraction slides if appropriate), belt pulleys, lathe motors, model trimmer, casting machine. These are not dental equipment but part of the office: door hinges, office chairs, typewriter, adding machine, duplicating machines, and so forth.

If you're not aware, many business machine outlets have what are known as "maintenance agreements" and their agents will come by on a regular predetermined schedule and perform the normal lubrication and maintenance for you. You should be aware, though, that these may pay for themselves if you utilize the machine a great deal. It would not really pay to buy a maintenance contract at say $30-$40 per year when you only use the machine one morning each month, and the machine only costs $300-$400 to start with. So be sure to discuss this with your doctor prior to agreeing to one.

If the doctor buys some new piece of equipment, say a typewriter, be sure to be there when the machine is delivered and set up. Have the installer go through its total maintenance with you and take notes. Record specifically where to oil and how. Also take note of when oiling (and cleaning) should take place. Then record the oiling dates in your regular maintenance calendar (you do have one, don't you?) and file the notes on the specific locations and directions for oiling in the master file under "equipment maintenance." This way the work can go on and the equipment will be properly cared for even if you are on vacation or (perish the thought—replaced).

We have been discussing oil, but in many places you will need grease. The prime difference is here you will usually apply it—still sparingly—at less frequent intervals. It will usually be applied at major wear areas on heavy equipment. An example would be the slide of a back rest on a dental chair. You must first clean off the old junk with a cloth that has been moistened with a cleaner. Remove all possible remnants of the old lubricant. It is not usually a clean job as the grease picks up dust and minute metal particles and gets pretty dark and dirty. If possible schedule things so that you will grease all the greaseable things in the office at the same time. Then don a pair of disposable plastic gloves and work in these.

Once the old stuff has been removed and all traces of the cleaner are wiped off, you can apply a thin film of the lubricant to the metal slides. There may be a specific brand recommended, but ordinary Vaseline works beautifully. Don't put too much on as it will have a tendency to pile up on the ends of the slide and may get smeared all over you, doctor and company.

Do not use any type of auto grease as all of these have specific odors and will tend to smell up the room.

One last word about lubrication—its main purpose is to reduce friction which will in turn make things run smoother and easier. It is your duty to help make everything easier for your doctor as well as yourself, so keep things well oiled. Don't hesitate to alter a set schedule and clean and oil something earlier if you find it binding ever so slightly. Sometimes a piece of equipment is used more than usual and needs more maintenance. Sometimes there is simply more dust in the atmosphere than normal and this will help to gum things up. And frankly sometimes things simply do not get as properly cleaned and oiled as they should have been and require earlier maintenance.

Are Your Instruments Sharp?

Little need be said here except that there is no excuse for your doctor having to use a dull instrument. A dull tool is little better than no tool at all. If it functions at all, your doctor will have to double or triple the amount of hand pressure and/or time in order to be effective. And this can only increase tension in the office. If kept up on a regular basis, the sharpening of instruments can be a quite minor task.

One major error when attempting to sharpen, say, a chisel is to alter the cutting angle. You are aware, of course, that each hand instrument is specifically and exactly made to conform with certain cutting angles. All sharpening must maintain these exact angles otherwise it will automatically become a different instrument!

If you are shapening by hand on an Arkansas stone, brace your free finger and hand so that the instrument can be always held at one angle with each pass down the stone. You will find this much easier to do if you allow yourself plenty of room on the bench or table and make major arm sweeps, keeping your fingers and hand steady and moving the arm at the shoulder. Look very closely at the cutting angle first and practice the movement a few times prior to actually letting the instrument touch the stone. It's quite easy to ruin an instrument with improper sharpening, so please use care.

If you find a great deal of difficulty in holding the correct angle, you can take a block of acrylic (make yourself one) and with a stone simply cut down grooves in it (label them) with the correct angle for the specific instruments. These grooves must be wide enough to permit some slide of the instrument as it sharpens, yet small enough to allow minimum play. You can then place the tool over the Arkansas stone, support it with the block and your finger and hone away safely and accurately. You'll need a different groove for each angle so you may need several blocks. Once made, however, they'll provide you with a lot of help.

This accuracy applies even more to the motorized sharpeners. In addition to ruining the cutting angle quickly, you can also heat up the tool and cause it to lose its temper and ability to maintain a sharp edge. The harder the metal, the sharper and more durable will be the cutting edge. If you heat it and let it cool slowly, it will have the effect of softening the metal—it will lose its "temper." So sharpening machines are geared down to relatively slow speeds to keep you from heating the tools excessively. Excessive pressure will increase the heat too, so don't bear down hard at any time.

If you are using a hand stone in a handpiece, be especially sure to turn it at a slow speed.

If you are not familiar with the way to sharpen a specific tool, have your doctor show you. It is better to take up some of his valuable time than to ruin a tool.

Set aside just a few minutes each week to sharpen instruments. Schedule it so you know in advance which ones to work on. You can judge this on their relative frequency of use (and relative quality). For instance, if the dentist uses a gingival margin trimmer no more than a couple of times a week, you will probably not need to sharpen this particular tool more frequently than every ten to twelve times used or maybe once a month, whereas he may use a biangle chisel several times daily. This latter tool would definitely need sharpening at least weekly.

If you find yourself spending seemingly excessive amounts of time sharpening tools and there is not other member of the team available to help you, you might suggest to the dentist that he purchase better instruments. These would be made with carbide steel tips which, although more expensive initially, will maintain their cutting edge longer and reduce maintenance time. In this way they quickly pay for themselves.

Burs wear out quickly, even when using carbide steel ones. This is due to the fact that enamel is so hard. Learn to feel each bur after its usage and determine whether or not it can be used again. On this ask your doctor to indicate to you just how each bur should feel before it is discarded. A dull bur will require more hand pressure, generate more heat and take longer to do its job. This has the effect of slowing things down and increasing doctor's tension, and it also increases more irritation to the dental pulp. A tooth that has been prepared with a dull bur will always be more sensitive to cold (and even to heat) the following day than one prepared with a sharp bur. Take time to consider the patient.

If your dentist abhors using a bur only once or twice and finding it too dull to use further, but too expensive to discard, save all of them. You can check your dental journals for ads from grinding companies that will regrind your old burs at a nominal cost. They will be returned as good as new but one number smaller. That is, if you send them a dull #557, you'll get back a sharp #556. You can thus recover some of the many you "wasted" and utilize the bur more efficiently.

Leather and Fabric Care

You are quite aware, I am sure, that one of your duties is the upkeep of the equipment and this applies naturally to the chair seats and covers. These will usually be vinyl if your chairs are of recent vintage, but could also be fabric (nylon or rayon) or even leather. The care of this material is important, though a relatively minor chore.

After weeks of usage your vinyl-covered chair may begin to show some spots where dirt has begun to accumulate. This will usually be in the small cracks and folds of the surface covering and will tend to give it a rather dingy look. You may dust it daily, but it will still occur, so you will need to clean it every once in a while. Cleaning is made easy these days by using one of the commercial liquid cleaners that are readily available. Some of these are heavily scented with pine oil, or lemon oil, and will smell up the office with a rather cheap and offensive odor, so stay away from these. All have some odor, so it's best to wait until the day it over, and keep a window open if possible before using the cleaner. Some of these type cleaners will need to be diluted so read the labels on the bottle carefully. If the one you use tends to leave a film when it dries, you'll have to wipe everything off again, which is wasted time, so find one that doesn't.

If you find some especially hard areas or deep folds that you cannot seem to get with a sponge, get a soft, multitufted toothbrush for gentle scrubbing.

If your chair is an older one and has real leather, buy some saddle soap at your local shoe shop or shoe store and following directions on the can, scrub it thoroughly with this. This tends to "freshen" and soften the leather in addition to cleaning it.

If you have fabric upholstery on your chair, go to a local furniture store and ask the manager to recommend to you the best fabric cleaner available in your area. These may vary from fabric to fabric so know ahead of time what your material is as well as the material used for stuffing the chair. Some internal materials may tend to gather into lumps when wet too much. You also need to know approximately how long it will take to dry, so you can plan your time accordingly. Note here also about the concern for odors.

Incidentally, if you simply find an individual spot or two of grime on the fabric, try one of the commercial "spot lifters." These are quite effective, especially for smaller areas, but once again watch the odors. There are ample chemical-type odors in the office as it is, so don't add any more than absolutely necessary.

Do not wax any type of material used in the seat, back, or leg rest. Number one, the wax just may cause early deterioration of the material (leather or vinyl) and number two, think of what a residue of wax might do to Mrs. Jones' expensive white linen suit. A third point is that the wax has a tendency to collect even more dust and grime.

Waxes Preserve Finishes

Do use wax liberally elsewhere around the office though. I would recommend its use on almost any hard finish you have in order to protect its finish and to keep it sparkling clean.

Here you should first use a good cleaner. I speak of the metal parts of the chair and base, the unit (if metal), the arm rests, the counter tops, dental light, etc. After you have thoroughly cleaned each item, and removed any lingering film, apply a good semipaste or liquid wax to the piece. Use it as liberally as necessary to cover completely, but not to the point where you are, as the TV commercials have said, "polishing the polish." With a thick coat of wax, you'll find that finishes will last longer. Paint will have less tendency to chip off or dull and fade.

One area that seems to deteriorate quickly is the arm rest. You should apply special attention here; patients tend to sweat a lot in the dental chair (for some peculiar reason!) and the arm rest and hand grip get a lot of moisture and sweat. This seems to pit and remove the high glaze from the bakelite-type arm rests so it is an excellent idea to keep a cloth moistened with liquid wax and lightly rub off the hard arm rests with this wax-dampened cloth between each patient. Do not leave a heavy excess as this will get on patients' hands and clothes. They will not appreciate this, of course, so if you can rub it with your finger and get any residue of wax at all, it is too much wax.

Many DAs use an alcohol sponge for this rubbing of the arm rests between patients (for antibacterial action), but this is really not necessary and tends to leave the rests spotty looking. The wax will do an ample job and preserve the finish much better.

Incidentally, in waxing the dental light, do not wax the lens or glass part, or the hand grips. Look at the lens between each patient and insure against spots of saliva or blood being splattered and left there. A water-moistened paper towel is usually sufficient for cleaning although a commerical window cleaning spray is also nice if you have time. The handles should be wiped with an alcohol sponge or sprayed with a spray-type disinfectant. Remember that the light gets hot and heat melts and cooks wax, so use it rather sparingly here. The same wax-moistened cloth you use for the arm rests will do the job nicely.

Now here is where efficiency must play an important part in your job. You have to wipe off various objects in the room between patients, and you have to use three different types of wipes—water, alcohol, and wax. Plan your movements so that you are as rapid and thorough as possible, as these wipings are necessary and important.

One procedure might be something like this—first wipe: the waxing cloth; secondly, wash your hands and wipe the light lens with the moistened paper towel (or cloth towel if you use them) with which you dried your hands. There is usually sufficient moisture left in them to do the job. Finally wipe the air and water syringe (and their carriages or holders) and any other parts of the chair you or the doctor might touch with contaminated hands with the alcohol syringe. Then (assuming you've already disposed of the old contaminated instruments, cups, burs, etc.) you're ready for seating the next patient.

Suction

The advent of the suction equipment in the dental office has certainly helped to speed things up. In fact, there are many, many offices that have to shut down if the suction goes on the blink. Naturally it must be kept in top-notch condition at all times.

One major problem is to prevent clogging of the suction apparatus with debris. This rule should apply: do not attempt to overwork the system. This means don't force it to pick up particles or matter too large for the tubes available. For instance, a piece of amalgam that is four millimeters by two millimeters may start into a hole (via the two millimeter side) that is three millimeters inside your suction tip, but get turned around and lodge somewhere inside via the four millimeter side. If it is still lodged when you pull in, say some hydrocolloid, you may well clog the entire system. Presumably it can be unclogged, but that will require time and this you do not have, especially while the patient is in the chair and the doctor is working. So, to repeat, don't force the system to overtax its capabilities.

Most saliva ejectors on units have small wire screen filters for collecting small bits of material that may clog the system. So what usually happens is that the screen itself becomes clogged. It is a simple enough procedure to unscrew the black rubber cap and remove the dirty screen, wash it out and replace it and start again, but it should never be allowed to accumulate debris to such an extent as to require cleaning during the day while patients are being seen. So set up a regular cleaning schedule for all the saliva ejector screens in the office—once a week, twice a week, or twice monthly—whatever you find necessary in order to eliminate any fear of clogging during the treatment of a patient.

Being realistic, occasionally it will clog while in the midst of treatment, requiring that you stop and clean it, but at least you've done every type of preventive measure possible.

Odor is a frequent and persistent problem in the office and stale and rotton saliva and tissue particles can be particularly offensive. These things accumulate from inadequate internal cleaning within the system. This means you simply must flush the evacuation system thoroughly between patients. If debris is allowed to dry on the inner surface of a pipe or tube you'll have a great deal of trouble getting it cleaned off. After each patient try to arrange to run clean water through the system for at least ten to twenty seconds. The important point is to keep the debris from drying, so if you have a long-extended patient and there is a likelihood of drying within the evacuation tubing before your doctor discharges the patient, try to find a moment or two to run fresh water through the system while the patient is still seated.

If you do find material has dried in the system, here's what to do: run fresh hot water through it for ten seconds or so, then turn the system off while still holding the tips in water, so that it shuts down with water in it if possible (and not the drying air). After five minutes, repeat this same procedure exactly. Then wait another five minutes. Usually three "softening" periods will be sufficient so that the first flushing with water will clear the tube of the dried matter.

Some commercially available evacuator system cleaners are available and contain specific chemicals for dissolving the matter, but fresh water in the prescribed manner will also work. The odor comes from the junk, so you really don't need deodorizer, just a clean system.

Disinfectants used within the system sound useful, but again are not really very helpful. Just a thoroughly washed system will usually suffice. If you wish, you can suck your old cold sterilizing solution through each system whenever you dispose of it, or use a commercial disinfectant, but their effectiveness has not been proven out over the long run. Just keep it simple and wash out the system with fresh water and you'll save time and money and still have an effective suction.

14

Increasing Efficiency in the Office Laboratory

Your Role in the Lab—Organization

In most dental offices that have any replacement service at all, the laboratory is a vital section. If your office is located such that a commercial dental laboratory is nearby, your duties may not amount to much, but many times your doctor has a lab in his suite and you must manage it properly. This area can become a tremendous bottleneck or it can be a real asset, depending on how you work with it and how you and your doctor have it organized.

Here is this key word again: *organization*. You must have a plan for every eventuality and be able to follow through accordingly. The purpose of the lab is, of course, to construct or alter or polish specific items in dentistry. It is the "kitchen." Just like the operatory, you must take note of every single piece of equipment and instrument and insure that it works properly at all times and is properly sharpened and has a specific place.

If your doctor happens to have a complete laboratory and employs a part- or full-time dental laboratory technician, you should have your doctor specifically spell out to both you and the lab technician each of your duties and responsibilities in the lab.

If there is not a technician, but a rather complete lab, you need to ascertain just how much lab work your doctor prefers that you do for him. If you or one of the other DAs in the office have time, it will certainly be a boon to the doctor if you can do some of the lab work. It is entirely possible that he may want or permit you to do total gold work there. This means pouring of the impressions and making of the dies, wax-ups, investing and casting as well as polishing. If you feel you are capable of any of this and have time and he has the equipment, you should certainly consider offering your services.

Usually he will need to repolish castings after intra-oral adjustments are made. It will usually only take three to five minutes, but you could easily do this for the doctor in the lab while he could be anesthetizing another patient, or changing a dressing or removing suctures, or even checking the hygienist's patient. The same could apply to the polishing of an adjusted periphery or occlusal surface of a denture adjustment.

Whatever laboratory work you finally do perform, be sure you take time to work through the procedures for maximum efficiency. In doing this set out every instrument, bur, wheel, brush, compound, pumice, tray, etc. that you'll need. Set them up in order of use and in such locations as to require minimal movement, and no searching for a single piece of equipment. Try to arrange the equipment in such a fashion as to require minimum movement or turning on your part.

In order to keep your polishing burs and brushes straight and in order, collect several of the small plastic containers that steel burs are packed in—they contain six holes or slots. Then find a shallow cardboard box and tape or glue these plastic containers to the bottom of the box in the lines or rows that you will want your burs. Next mix an amount of plaster and pour it into the box to a thickness of about one-quarter inch. After it sets completely, you can peel the cardboard away (it will be easy if it's still damp), and you'll have a customized bur block specifically for lab burs. The advantage here is that you can space the bur holders as far apart as you need to in order to give yourself plenty of room for brushes, large stones, wheels, and the like: Usually you can accomplish it all with a bur block no more than 2 x 4 inches. You may find it helpful to take a pencil and scribe in the set plaster each bur number or "brush," "wheel," "white stone," or "green stone," etc., so you'll know, or anyone else will know exactly where everything goes. In addition, you'll know exactly what is missing if something isn't replaced as it should be.

If you use the cloth and chamois wheels on a dental lathe, you should try to arrange it so you can have a small panel or board with some nails or pins sticking out. On these pins you can quickly slip a rag wheel or polishing wheel. If you work beside a cabinet with a hinged door, you can frequently place these wheels on the inside of the door. Then you simply work with the cabinet door open and the wheels exposed and readily accessible. After use, the door can be closed and the wheels moved out of sight and clutter. If you do this, however, I recommend painting the back of the door behind the wheels a dark color, since the polishing compound will smudge the paint and it will always look dirty. (This is one area you'll find nearly impossible to keep clean.)

If you do much polishing and grinding of gold in the lab, be sure to get a "catch pan." This is simply a shallow pan—maybe 8 x 12 inches, with a piece of clear plastic, plexiglas, celluloid, etc. curved broadly over the top to a height of perhaps 8 inches. You do all of your grinding in this pan by inserting one hand holding the casting in one side, and the handpiece and bur in the other. All grindings are therefore collected. At the end of a year, these gold chips can be sent in to a smelting company and exchanged for more gold ingots or money. It can frequently amount to several hundred dollars. It is quite easy to make such a pan, or your dealer can sell you one.

Incidentally, if your doctor does much hand grinding at the chair, why not provide him one for usage there. It could be set on the bracket table or cervical tray or even counter within easy reach of both his hands and he could save a great of gold and money here, too. If it seems like too much trouble or wasted motion for him to use the catch pan, don't bother. The time wasted will never be caught up by the savings of the gold; time is more valuable than gold in the busy dental office.

If you frequently need to change from polishing compound and rouge to pumice and chalk and back again, you'll probably be better off having duplicate splash pans, one for pumice, etc., the other for compound and rouge. You will save time just by switching pans rather than by washing it out again to go back to compound.

Cleanliness Is Next to . . .

Since most of the work being performed in the lab is more or less "dirty" work, it frequently becomes the dirtiest room in the suite. Certainly many dentists when proudly showing off their dental office, rather hurriedly open and shut the laboratory door—ashamed of its dust, its dirty, cluttered appearance. We all realize that water gets splashed, plaster spills and tracks the floor, waxes drop on floors and get smeared, and rag wheel strings fly around the lab, but we all also know that the lab simply must be kept clean. Like it or not, time consuming or not, it behooves the dental assistant to keep the lab clean. If for no other reason, the lab can be a breaking point in the sterility of an office procedure. You and your doctor carefully wash your hands in front of the patient. Do you sterilize instruments, hand syringes, and equipment, then take a casting to a lab and contaminate it? I hope not. It would be like dining at the most exclusive restaurant in town, where the tableware and even the waiters are spotless, the very epitome of real "class," then opening the door to the kitchen and it looks like the behind-the-counter of a "greasy-spoon" skid row diner. Is this your office? Remember, the only health inspector is your own conscience. Is your conscience clean?

Keep a moistened sponge near the sink. Any time there is even a slight spill or splatter, wipe it up as soon as it occurs. If some plaster spills, for heaven's sake wipe it up then. If possible get a small sized portable vacuum cleaner and keep it handy in the lab. If you have central suction in the office, you may want to use this to suction up the spilled plaster, but it would be better not to. Remember the suction carries moisture and if you get any plaster set up in your system, you will have a major repair and expense on your hands. If you should get any dry plaster into the system, be certain to run a great deal of water through it so as to try to flush all of the plaster through the system before it has an opportunity to set up within.

If wax spills on the floor, scrape it up as soon as possible.

Then moisten a sponge with a wax solvent and lightly wipe off the remaining film. Remember, the solvent may also dissolve certain kinds of varnishes or types of flooring panels, so use it sparingly.

If your doctor runs the lathe frequently, you'll usually find the lab accumulates a lot of dust. Your doctor can purchase a vacuum attachment for the lathe which will help, but you'll still get the dust accumulation. Your only other recourse is to dust as frequently as possible. A suggestion would be to do strip or spot dusting. This is to regularly keep a dust cloth out on a bench near the door to the lab. Then every time you walk in and have a free hand (I realize you'll not always have a free hand) grab the cloth and dust something. Dust the model trimmer once, then the lathe, then the bench engine, then the desk lamp, then the counter top in one spot, then another, and so on. If you follow this step-wise method, you'll keep things under close enough control to at least keep the lab respectable during the day. Then you can hopefully spend a minimum amount of time once daily for complete dusting.

As you pour models or impressions, get some six-inch squares of glass or plexiglas and "plop" the poured impressions on these. Then you can set these aside—even inside the cabinet for final setting and they will be neat and out of the way.

How to Schedule the Commercial Laboratories

In the trials and tribulations of the average day, nothing is quite so frustrating as to find that the twenty-unit bridge for Mrs. Pesky is not back from the lab. You call the lab and they say this or that, but the basic fact remains that it's simply not ready yet. This is a problem we all face from time to time, but certainly every effort must be made to overcome it.

If you consistently receive work late from the lab, you should call them and see if you can iron out the problem. Perhaps you are not allowing ample working time. If there is no improvement, you might suggest to your doctor that he change labs. If he declines to do this, why not mark on the lab slip a due date one or two days prior to the actual date you need the bridge? If you do this, you should note a couple of things. Do not mark down a due date for a day on which you are not working, such as a Sunday or a holiday. Also you should be consistent and if you should call the lab about the bridge and they should happen to casually ask you for the due date, you might give yourself away if you mentioned the true date. If the lab once got the notion that you were predating their work, you'd probably continue getting the work back a day later.

There is a sort of axiom that goes something like this: "If you call the lab and scream louder than the other guy, the lab will set his work aside and do yours." This is a pretty crude way to put it, but frankly has proven effective many times. It simply means that many labs, particularly smaller ones, will respond more quickly to the maximum pressure. If you hound them and gripe more about the lousy service, they'll likely try harder to please and give you better service than the office that accepts quietly anything they give it. If you do decide to follow this practice, please try to use it strictly as a last resort. We need all the good relations between dental office and dental laboratory we can get.

In order to get the best service from the labs, try to cooperate with them. In this I suggest the following: have concise, clear, and legible work orders. If there is a critical shading problem, send a shade guide along. Incidentally, if you doctor has not heard of the Jelenko "Shade-a-Guide," you might recommend it to him. You simply paint onto a conventional shade guide special stains or shades to match exactly what you want. You send in the touched-up shade guide for the lab to match exactly. This eliminates guesswork and then the special stains can be cleaned off of the guide when it returns from the lab for further usage.

Have impressions as sharp as possible. Remember, the casting will be no more accurate than the impressions. On this point, you'd better let your dentist make the decision about what to send to the lab.

If you are pouring the impression and trimming dies, etc., don't waste time and let them sit around the office very long. In the first place they take up room and clutter up the office, and in the second place, give the lab as much time to work as possible.

This will help everyone: get a set of 3 x 5 file cards and keep a record and critique of each piece of work you get back from the

```
┌─────────────────────────────────────────────────────────────┐
│                                                               │
│   To the Laboratory: Jones Dental Studio                      │
│   Case: Smiyhe                    Date: 2-17-72               │
│   Item: Four-unit Ceramco Bridge                              │
│   Notes:   too high in occlusion                              │
│            poor axial contours                                │
│            excellent shade matching                           │
│                                          Dr. I. M. Sample     │
│                                                               │
└─────────────────────────────────────────────────────────────┘
```

Figure 14-1:   Laboratory Criticism Card

lab (see Figure 14-1). Ask the doctor to tell you what he likes and dislikes about each thing and then you keep this on file in the office. Tell the lab about each piece so they can work accordingly. It just might be they think they are pleasing the dentist, when in reality they could be doing something he would like better.

Keep a carbon copy of all laboratory work orders. In this way you can refer to it and know exactly what you told the lab if there's any comeback at all from them.

If it is necessary that you mail things to the lab, keep a close record on how long mail delivery takes to and from the lab. Be sure to allow extra time over holidays. If you send a self-addressed card along, the lab can mail it back to you with their anticipated mailing date on it so you can schedule your patients accordingly.

You or the secretary should keep a chalkboard in the lab and record on it each patient's name for whom you are expecting lab work. Record the due date (actual) and the initial of the lab to which the work was sent. Keep a calendar nearby. Then each day you check off whether or not the work has been received for the patient due the following day. If it has not been received, you promptly get on the telephone and inquire about it. You will course, rub off the patient's name following insertion of the appliance or casting. In this way you will have a simple, efficient and convenient method of keeping in touch with the lab work.

part 3

The Dental
Hygienist

15

Developing Hygienic Efficiency in Your Area

Isn't a Prophy a Prophy?

To paraphrase an old saying, "A prophy is a prophy is a prophy." Isn't it? In reality, you, the qualified dental hygienist, and I, the dentist, know it just is not so. There are the easy, light prophies that reveal no calculus and practically no plaque or stain, and then there is Mr. Blackmouth, the pipe smoker, who declines to have his teeth cleaned until they are totally covered with coal tar. It just isn't quite the same thing, is it? Yet frequently the dental secretary doesn't know or realize this fact and she schedules Miss Prettyteeth and Mr. Blackmouth for equal length appointments. You finish Miss Prettyteeth in fifteen minutes and have maybe a half-hour to go over home care, which seems rather absurd since she does all of her home care as perfectly as we do. Wasted time.

Then you get Mr. Blackmouth and just barely finish one quadrant when your time runs out. And invariably he is "too busy" to keep coming back for more visits and complains you're too slow—that the "girl" in another office he went to one time finished in half an hour. (He failed to mention or realize that she only used coarse pumice and did not perform subgingival scaling. She only polished the top of the iceberg.)

In other words, some patients simply need much more time for manual treatment as well as oral instruction than do others. This information must be obtained and passed on to the appointment secretary if you are to render optimal service to all of your patients. You must always have ample time, but no excess time allotted.

An interesting point comes when you see a patient who has not seen a dentist for several years and in reality needs periodontal treatment instead of a "routine" prophylaxis. Yet, here she is scheduled with you. Should you go ahead and perform a prophy or just call the dentist for his evaluation and probable rescheduling? You should try to prearrange such happenings with your dentist and know his opinions first. Sit down and discuss it with him.

If a patient needs periodontal treatment severely, a "prophy" isn't going to help much. You simply will not be able to scale deeply enough into the pockets to be very effective. True you can effect some gingival shrinkage and polish the "stains and accretions" off of the teeth, but the real damage-producing matter is farther subgingival than most state boards permit you to go. If you do penetrate far down, you are in reality moving into the realm of periodontal disease treatment which is "dentistry," not "dental hygiene." So, it can be a touchy subject, bordering on one with legal implications, and you'd better iron it out thoroughly with your dentist prior to much deep subgingival scaling and curettage.

How to See More Patients in Less Time

Just as a great amount of time and effort are spent making the dentist more efficient, the same applies to the dental hygienist. Your capacity as an income producer in the office make you quite a valuable individual. It therefore behooves you to concentrate on being as efficient as possible, and you can pretty well follow the steps of the dentist.

Try preset trays. Have several trays already arranged with exactly the instruments you'll need on them—in order.

You should concentrate on making all of your prophies as systematic as possible. That is, start with a certain instrument of your choice every time and use it completely until you can discard it. Do everything with that particular tool that you can before you lay it aside. Then do the same with the next. Each time you have to lay an instrument down and search for and pick up another, you lose time.

Start in the same area on every patient, say the maxillary right third molar. If you are starting with, say, a curette, proceed from the distal of the third molar, to the facial to the mesial, then the distal, facial, mesial, and so on to the distal of the upper left third molar. Then come back with this same tool on all of the linguals from the distal, lingual, mesial, distal, lingual, mesial aspect of the upper left third, second and so on. Then start on the mandible in the same fashion.

Next follow on through with the next instrument of your choice, say a scaler, and follow the same type of cycle around the mouth. In this manner you can usually make no more than two cycles around the mouth for complete scaling, and you'll only change instruments once.

If you find you cannot get to certain areas for thorough scaling on one of your circuits and will need another specific tool, don't stop at that moment and get it, use it, then go back to your original starting tool, but make a mental note and remember the area(s) in question and just exactly which tool you will need and where you will find it if it is stored in your dental cabinet. After you finish your cycle, you may find additional problem areas and you can catch these all (in cycle fashion) with the same instrument instead of constantly switching.

It will prove quite beneficial to you also if you utilize double-ended instruments. This will enable you to get nearly all areas of the mouth with one instrument—using both ends, which will save time in picking up and switching, in addition to cleaning and sterilizing time later. If you will shop around, you can frequently find mixed ends, say a scaler on one end and a curette on the other. Certain manufacturers will provide you with such also, at slight additional cost. You also may be interested in instruments with changeable tips. With these you can add whichever tips you wish and strictly customize your instruments.

When you are scaling or polishing, a great deal of time is lost permitting the patient to empty his mouth and rinse. Elimination, or at least reduction of this, will save you enormous amounts of time. Let's face it though, there are times when *you* want to rid the mouth of saliva and/or blood, so you should at least work with a comfortable saliva ejector constantly or preferably a high-velocity evacuation tip. You can purchase various types of tips that will evacuate the mouth, and retract the tongue from your way, and yet permit ample room for your fingers and instruments. Your dental supply house detail man can help you with this.

A point of advice here when you do not intend to permit the patient to stop and rinse is to beat him to the punch. That is, if you tell him in advance that you will "stop in a few minutes to let him rinse," he'll much more likely sit patiently and let you work, than if you say nothing and he feels you are not concerned. In this instance he will probably interrupt you so he can rinse. It is important that you remain in control.

As you are polishing you will probably find it convenient to use a finger cup dispenser for the pumice. In this manner you need only move your hand and handpiece three inches for more pumice instead of a foot or two to the bracket table or even cervical tray. If you utilize pumice and then chalk, you can use a double finger cup.

Many companies provide premixed, premeasured pumice and/or chalk and these are sometimes helpful and save setting-up time and clean-up time if you like the results or brands. These are generally slightly more costly, so if you prefer to buy in bulk which is cheaper, you should consider buying also small disposable aluminum foil-coated paper cups (about one inch in diameter and height) and every week or so preload a number of these. They will fit into a thumb cup and are completely disposable.

It's usually convenient to keep a sponge or a tissue in your hand with the thumb cup for wiping of the rubber polishing cup as you progress. Many hygienists use a napkin or tissue pinned to the bib, but this is a longer distance away from the mouth than your hand, so would take more time. Besides it occasionally happens that the moisture on the wipe will seep through even the bib and wet the patient's clothing.

If you have a patient with exceedingly heavy stain, you'll probably want to add some of the commercial stain removing or "ex-tar" type of pumice compounds to your regular polishing agents. If you find none of these available, at least add some coarse pumice, which will remove the heavy tar pretty well. Please be sure to go over the teeth with polishing chalk after using these coarse, heavy-duty type polishers, however, because they tend to roughen and scratch the enamel.

If you have one of the ultrasonic scalers available, be sure to use ample water spray to reduce the heat and discomfort. You'll probably find it advantageous to tilt the patient back farther when using this apparatus. This tends to bring the tongue up over the throat automatically and creates less tendency to swallow and/or choke on the part of the patient. Naturally a high-speed suction is mandatory. Again try to adapt your technique so that you are required to change tips a bare minimum of times.

If you do not have the ultrasonic equipment available, but have a high-speed handpiece, you can order some special friction grip burs for it which will create almost the same effect as the ultrasonic scalers. These burs are specially designed to bump against the calculus and tooth surface and "vibrate" it clean. There are two types—a larger, bulk type and a smaller, more pointed one for subgingival scaling. Both are very effective and quite economical, but extreme care in handling must be utilized as they can "notch" the cementum or dentin if you apply too much pressure. Steady water flow on the tip is used as with all ultrasonic equipment, so suction is necessary.

If you find yourself with a patient like Mr. Blackmouth, you'll know as soon as he opens his mouth. This is the time to point out to him that his mouth is in such a state as to require at least two, maybe three appointments for complete treatment. In this way he will not be so concerned when after, say three-quarters of an hour, when your fingers are about to break off, you tell him you'll need him back again. He will not get the idea you're quitting just because you're tired or because you have another patient to see. It is always best to anticipate and tell him in advance. If you should happen to find things easier than you thought and finish, so much the better, and you can make him feel good when you tell him it wasn't as hard as it looked.

Whenever you do see a Miss Cleantooth, do everything you possibly can to impress on her that she needs to become a "missionary" for good dental health. These people seem to be so few and far between that they must be made as knowledgeable about our problems as possible. Tell her about other patients like Mr. Blackmouth (no names, of course) and how it would be so nice if she and others like her could go out and simply be enthusiastic about good home care and dental health to their friends.

Where and How to Find Literature

As you are aware, part of your job is dental education. In fact, it becomes more and more important in these days of emphasis on prevention. You can talk and talk during your sessions with your patients, and they will frequently listen and understand, but they also have a tendency to forget little details here and there. For this reason it is quite helpful to have plenty of dental educational literature available to send home with the patients. It is available from various sources—some free, some costly.

The free literature available is usually simple propaganda provided by commercial interests like toothpaste or toothbrush manufacturers. Nearly all of the major companies provide it for the asking. It is usually well-written, nicely printed, but on the last page will have some of their advertising. There is nothing really wrong with using this type of literature, but I would suggest that if you do, you point out that it is provided by a commercial company and that you do not specifically recommend this and only this product. They simply provided some suitable pamphlets.

Somewhat less commercialized and quite good is literature provided by many state dairy associations. Their work frequently is free and discuss dietary needs and dentistry. These are commercial only in the sense of the "association" and not a specific corporation.

Some state public health departments provide free dental literature—especially for school use, but also available for distribution to the profession.

A number of printing houses around the country have excellent literature available at nominal costs. It can add your dentist's name on the bottom if he should desire.

It is generally considered best if you have your own individual literature printed. In this way you say what you want to say, in your own words, and there is absolutely no commercialism connected with it.

A point: if you do choose to dispense any literature at all, be sure to read it carefully first. Make certain it says what you would say and does not say something that you disagree with. Some of this literature is apparently written by writers and not by dental authorities and may not always be 100 percent accurate.

If you prepare your own literature, you must first let your dentist edit it. After all it's his name and office that it is going out under and you must make sure he agrees with everything you say.

Once you have it all written and okayed, I would suggest you present it to an offset printer. He can make a "plate" and you can have additional copies run at any time, at a minimal cost without having to reset the type. Remember though that if you want to change any wording, you'll need to discard that plate and start over.

Incidentally, it is a good idea to read over your literature every year or so. Ideas change and you may be passing out literature with old and outdated suggestions and instructions in it.

The Better Home Care

Speaking of dental literature, thousands upon thousands of reams of paper have been applied to home instructions for patients, and uncountable words have been said—much of it to little or no avail. All too frequently the patient simply nods his head in seeming acknowledgment, and then he goes home and does about what he had been doing before. Pretty disillusioning, isn't it?

Well the major difficulty is probably that things are a little too "rote." Too, too routine. The secret is to really let the patient know (not just think, but *know*) that *this* home care instruction is for him alone. It will not necessarily work for his wife or children or parents, but you feel it will work for him. In other words, you have customized his home care and you make certain he knows it.

He has heard for years to "brush the teeth the way they grow," or "back and forth," or "up and down." And quite frequently this is reasonably satisfactory for the mass public, but now you must break it down to a specific individual.

As you progress through his prophy you must take note of specific problem areas of his mouth. Such areas are difficult enough for you to reach, so you can well imagine the difficulty he might have. These areas might be caused by missing teeth, or particularly malaligned teeth with deepened or narrow interdental spaces. He may have upper second or third molars or even lower seconds or thirds that require special positions of his mandible and tongue or cheeks in order to have access with a toothbrush.

A suggestion would be to start off the appointment for the regular routine prophylaxis by staining his entire mouth with disclosing solution. As you do so, tell him why you are doing this and what it will show (plaque). Then have him hold a hand mirror and you use a mouth mirror and point by point, go around his mouth and show him the "red" areas of plaque. It is a good idea to take an ordinary wooden toothpick and remove some stained plaque for him. This is preferable to using an explorer because he may feel the metal instrument simple does a better job of removing than anything he might have at home. Then proceed with your prophy in your conventional manner. I feel it is excellent technique to discuss plaque and all its aspects while performing the prophy. So especially point out that the plaque you have stained is primarily *yesterday's* food. He will probably think to himself, "Well, I ate a snack before coming here and they were clean before that." Note that it takes about twenty-four hours for plaque to form.

After you have finished your polishing, again hand him a hand mirror and using a sterilized toothbrush show him how the brush needs to be held and what he must do with his lower jaw and related structures in order to manipulate the brush adequately. (You may wish to give each patient a new one to take home, but it's best to emphasize you are recommending a "type," not a specific brand.) And then let him watch you move the bristles into each problem area. Then hand him the toothbrush and let him show you (and himself) how well he can preform with it. Ask him if he feels he can reach every area adequately.

If he has particular difficulty in reaching certain areas with the brush, you may feel it helpful to teach him to use one of the so called "perio-aids" which are plastic holders for short round toothpick tips. Teach him how to chew the point of the toothpick slightly in order to sort of make a "bristle brush." Then he can direct the tip just about any spot in his mouth with more convenience than a regular brush.

You can show him the unwaxed floss technique if you feel he is ready for it.

The entire point of this is that he should be made to know and realize that he and only he will be able to benefit from this type of home care. You have taken specific time and effort to demonstrate to him the proper home care for him, and not just repeated an old speech. He is surely going to be more impressed and much more likely to follow through.

16 General Guidelines for Greater Success with Patients

How to Get Your Patients Enthusiastic About Home Care

No matter how much time and effort you put into it, quite frequently you simply work and work on training the patient on his home care, but the patient quickly loses his enthusiasm and drifts back into his old neglectful habits. The key to success is to let the patient truly know just how effective his own personal home care can be.

The way to go about this is to find an area in his mouth, say, an interdental papilla or two on his lower incisor area, that is reddened and swollen. Then point out to him the difference between this area and one that is normal. If necessary, show him close up part of your own mouth or even one of the other auxiliaries if there is one convenient. (The other DAs would certainly need to be briefed in advance about this possibility.)

Once he gets the idea of what a normal and an abnormal area look like, you can then proceed to coach him (with the face mirror) some specific method of your choice, say using the perio-aid and toothpick tip, and let him clean the affected area as prescribed for seven consecutive days. After that time have him return and you and he can both look and see that the area is in better shape—in fact, if he has followed through, it should look practically normal. If this doesn't impress your patient, no amount of talking is likely to.

It is important that you explain in advance what your plans are and what results he should expect to see. He must be shown and clearly taught what an inflammed section of gingiva looks like and the difference between that and normal. It may well be that he has always looked at his reddened, puffy gums and thought that they were normal. As you are aware, a surprisingly large number of patients do think bleeding gums are normal. If you can teach them the difference between normal and diseased, you will automatically create an enthusiasm that will not stop. No rational person will enjoy poor health if he is once shown what good health is and how to attain it.

If you attempt to show the average patient a mouth full of disease and compare it with a healthy one, it just might be too much to see. You could relate this to not seeing the trees for the forest. This is the main reason for picking out just one small spot and having him work only on this area at first. He must prove to himself that good home care—even if it is simple—can correct a diseased area. And if you can once convince a patient in his own mind how effective this can be, you've helped him acquire a lifetime of better-than-average dental health. He will appreciate you for it, and just think how nice it would be to only work in clean mouths!

Using the Audiovisual

If your office has audiovisual equipment available, you should certainly want to utilize it to its fullest advantage. It is for patient education and re-education and not just something to play with or stick off in a corner somewhere. If you have ever told a story to someone for the thousandth time, you might realize that occasionally you forget what you intended to say or leave some key phrase or item out. It might also occur to you to draw a diagram from time to time and you realize halfway through that your artistry isn't as good as your dental abilities. The AV takes care of all of this for you. It tells the same story or stories time after time, always exactly the same and has fine photographs or diagrams or drawings to match. And in color too.

The problem with most AVs is that the office staff doesn't usually use it wholeheartedly. It must become a regular, everyday thing, as routine as washing your hands, if it is to be effective. It must be just a matter of fact that the patients are to see the AVs.

Most of the various commercially made AVs are quite good and take about eight to ten minutes. Your doctor has no doubt selected those subjects he likes and feels comfortable with, but if you see one or two additional strips you prefer, there should be no harm in asking him to audition and hopefully, buy them. After all, your work with them is important and proper utilization of the machine is helpful.

You and the entire staff should sit down and go over the various subjects you have. Take them title by title and plan how they are to be shown to the patients. Certain films may be more of an advantage shown before the patient is treated, whereas others may be better for follow-up after treatment. Do not just lightly decide this as some films may have a tendency to confuse or even frighten a patient before a specific treatment. You or the dentist should briefly explain the procedure to the patient, perform it, then afterward show the AV to clarify any remaining questions. Remember, the more dentally educated your patient is, the better and more cooperative he will be. After he has viewed the film or filmstrip, you (or the DA) should always try to ask if there are any further questions. There rarely will be by this time.

Some patients are in quite a hurry to leave after arising from the chair, so always make sure they know you expect them to stay ten minutes longer. It should be more or less spelled out in the appointment schedule they receive.

The little General Electric "Show 'n Tell" audiovisual machine has proved quite valuable in many offices. Considering its price—under $50 complete—it's possibly one of your best bargains. It is certainly bordering on a toy in looks and somewhat in action, yet it provides roughly a three-minute story about certain vital phases of dentistry. There is a short filmstrip and a small record that plays simultaneously along with it. The record has one side labeled "Child" and is strictly geared to describe the filmstrip scene in terms a child can understand and appreciate. The other side of the record is labeled "Adult" and using the same filmstrip describes the actions on an adult level.

The real beauty of it is that when using it for children, the story is short enough to be readily accepted within their attention span. They listen to every word. Incidentally, if you are giving a fluoride treatment and need to time the activity for about four minutes, it works out just about perfectly if you (1) insert the gel, (2) get out the record and strip and begin playing, (3) let the story run to completion, (4) replace the record and strip in the case, and (5) remove the cotton rolls or "geltainers." The child watches the show, learns something, and gets a fluoride treatment without severe complaints. Works like a charm. You'll probably have to darken the room so the show can be seen better, so casually warn the child you will "dim" the lights and show a "movie."

Some doctors prefer to make up their own AVs, using slides made there in their own office and tape a background audio to them. This can then be set up on a slide projector and produces a very nice personalized program. It takes a little time to get the proper slide collection and the whole thing organized, but it usually listened to more attentively by the patients since it is their own dentist's voice they are listening to.

If you would like to compose such a show for specific aspects of dental hygiene, using your voice, I'm sure you doctor can quickly gather slide materials of ample sufficiency. It does require somewhat special equipment, however, which can run into a few dollars. You need a Kodak "Carousel" slide projector or something comparable that can be set to automatically flip to the next slide every ten, twelve, fourteen or so seconds. Then you need a tape player, preferably one that plays a cartridge (for simplicity and convenience).

Now you need to sit down and compose your "story"—what you want to say. You should limit it to a maximum length of ten minutes, because of the average patient's attention span dwindles after eight to ten minutes.

Now judge just where slides would be appropriate. You may, for instance, want to show normal gingiva, several angles or shots of different types of normal, then show various degrees of diseased gingiva. You may show a sequence of several days of home care on specific patients and each day's result—start to finish. You might also want to add shots or toothbrush positions, and usage of the various types of auxiliary aids—the "Stimudent," "perio-aid," "Denticator," rubber cup massage, finger massage. You certainly might want to add various shots of using unwaxed floss.

Next you recompose your story to fit the slides, then set it up on the sequencing projector and without recording, learn how to space out your dialogue. This is a very time-consuming procedure, but important. Once you have your timing down pat, run through the sequenced slides and record the story, and you are all set.

A word of caution: in order to have the show run normally, without your being there, it is important to be able to start both the projector and the tape player at the same time. Otherwise your slides may sequence differently from your voice and you'll lose the whole show. It is advisable to allow a few seconds before and after each slide is flipped before beginning your audio about that slide. This will permit a little buffer zone to catch up if the projector and recorder do not get properly sequenced—the show could still go on.

When and How to Utilize the "Take Homes"

I discussed where to get the "take home" literature in chapter 15, but it is very important to use them correctly if they are to be of any help at all. Again, the emphasis is on patient education, so the patient must read this material to benefit from it. You must persuade your patient to take the time to read it when he gets home.

First, I would recommend that you catalog all of the literature you have available. You may do this alphabetically or numerically depending on the number of different titles or subjects you have. Make a list of this cataloging and keep all of the literature bulk stored in as much the same order as you've cataloged as possible. Try to set up a cabinet drawer or file in your treatment room with maybe half a dozen pieces of each type handy to your fingertips. As has been mentioned earlier, know what your educational literature says and by all means, keep it current.

Now, as you perform your prophylaxis and run through various conversations about dentistry with your patient, keep a mental note on which particular subjects you covered. Then, at the end of the session, you can pull out specific pieces of literature and give this to the patient to take home. You should point out to him that the literature you are giving him will explain things you've been discussing in more detail and should help him more. Tell him if he has any further questions about the subject after reading the pamphlet(s) to be sure to call you or the doctor and you will be glad to explain further.

A really nice gesture, especially if you are giving out several different pieces to the same patient, is to have a standard manila envelope available, and write the patient's name on it and enclose all the literature in this. Many doctors do this with written copies of a treatment plan for the patient, in addition to enclosing some of the same educational material with it. (Some of these dentists have their own name preprinted on the outside of the manila folder and pick up a little free "name spreading" as the patient walks down the street carrying the oversized folder.) Anyway, it is a nice thing, and the patients seem to appreciate it and pay a little more heed to the importance of the literature.

If you have noticed that a particular patient needs some sort of dentistry, say a fixed bridge, and has failed to respond to your dentist's recommendation, you may want to casually slip in "fixed bridge" literature along with all the rest. It may be best not to mention anything about it, just let it appear when the patient opens the folder at home.

It is probably rather obvious that you will not want to send literature home with every patient. Some are just not receptable to it, and there is enough waste paper scattered around the landscape as it is. So be selective, and you'll find a practice of better and better patients month after month, year after year.

part 4

Administration of the Dental Office

17 Capitalizing on an Effective Office Manual

Why Should Your Office Have One?

In any dental office that has more than one dental auxiliary, there tends to be a separation of duties. That is, one person usually "runs" the desk and another "runs" the chair. A third assistant may have duties that overlap both of these sections, plus perhaps the laboratory. Then there is the dental hygientist who might possibly have a touch of all of the above-mentioned sections. Inevitably there is some overlapping of duties, and all too frequently there tends to be some personality involvement.

If one person, say, the dental secretary, has more or less been assigned certain specific duties, she knows she is solely responsible for these. She may set up a system of her own because it specifically suits her and works well for her. But then another auxiliary of the office comes in and perhaps doesn't understand the system and criticizes, and ill feelings are likely to result.

In addition, the doctor may walk in and not understand the system himself. Naturally it is imperative that he knows everything going on in the office, so this could be quite embarrassing to all concerned.

A problem frequently arises when one member of the staff is out—ill, day off, vacation, or what have you. Then the work load must be covered by others, and "private" systems—unknown by others, may be quite chaotic.

If the work load becomes overbearing, say at the chair, the hygienist or the secretary may need to be called in to assist temporarily, and it behooves these people to know how to "pick up the slack."

Then, too, there is the specific chore or duty that lies in that "gray area," with no specific assignment as to whom it should be done by. Who should do it? Are you going to argue about it? Ill feelings? Wasted time? Inefficiency?

The only real solution to these types of problems is to create for yourself or your office an office manual. Some offices call it a training manual, others a duty manual, but it is a book that spells out every conceivable duty and chore in the office and the responsibilities of each party. When speaking of this latter subject, I mean responsibilities of each dental auxiliary to the office and to each other, and of the doctor to the staff.

The manual will not be something you can build overnight or over a weekend—it will take months, but once it is operational you'll find your entire team functions better and more smoothly.

Problems to Be Overcome First

In the average overworked dental office, time is of the essence. There is simply no spare time to tackle something this big. Therefore, you all must resolve to spend an evening a week, or every other week, working on the manual. You may find it convenient to assign specific parts of it which can be done in group sessions.

Many subjects will be purely technical, and should create no real problems, but many will need major policy decisions by the dentist. He will need to be consulted from the very beginning, and will need to go along with the project, or else it will not be as helpful as it can be.

You should have an office conference one afternoon or evening and simply discuss what you want the manual to be like.

Remember that the doctor is the only truly permanent member of the office (and the boss), so his decisions will be needed and adhered to religiously. If he sets a policy you do not like, go ahead and record it if he insists, but you can try later to alter it. Policies can be changed, but it is his office and he will run it to his satisfaction, not necessarily yours or others on the staff.

In this conference you will need to mutually decide what you want in the manual and how you will want to set it up. You will want to define specific sections. These may be (1) General Office Policies, (2) Secretarial Duties, (3) Chairside Duties, (4) Rover's Duties, (5) Hygienist's Duties, (6) Miscellaneous.

Now you should take each section and mutually plan what goes there. The doctor will probably have the major amount of work in the "policy" section. He should sit down and spell out his thoughts, philosophy, aims, and expectations of his practice as related to the auxiliaries. He should specifically spell out the employment policies, such as hours, holidays, sick leave, vacation, uniforms, smoking privileges and so forth. This section alone will prove very helpful, for then there will be no questions on either side if there is any employment disagreement.

He should describe more or less how he wants to accept and handle new patients.

He needs to point out his preferences when patients fail to follow through with their obligations—financial as well as dental.

So far as the rest of the personnel are concerned, you should each plan to sit down and spell out in detail each task you have to do, and how you go about it. You should include enough detail so that a relatively untrained individual could read it and pretty much know what to do and how to do it. (By untrained, I mean another auxiliary who has not performed your specific job.)

You should spell out such specifics as how to go about filling out a bank or credit card, charge slip (if appropriate), and where the slips are kept, and the phone number of the bank if it is necessary to call, and how to handle the deposit slips thereafter. You should even go into detail with specific information as to where the slips are stored, before and after use, and what to do if they should all be used up.

In other words, every item or procedure in the entire office will need to be clearly spelled out. In this way if the secretary is out sick, the rover or chairside assistant could (with the aid of the manual) simply take over and do the work for her. This same step-by-step write-out should be done for each task of all of the auxiliaries, including the hygienist. True, the DA cannot substitute for the hygienist, but a substitute, temporary hygienist could use the manual and become a part of the team quickly. Remember, training someone takes the time of two people, the one learning and the one teaching, and the less time required by the teacher, the better, because she is needed elsewhere.

As may be obvious to you at this point, the manual is also a tremendous benefit to the doctor if he has to replace someone on the staff. He simply hands the new assistant the manual, and in a very short time, he has an efficient team again. You should not begrudge the fact that you may be preparing a training manual for your own replacement. If you like your job and your employer, you will take pride in your ability to help him; if you continue to perform well, you'll keep your job anyway.

How to Begin

Once you have had several planning sessions and know pretty clearly what you all want to do, you must set out to actually put it together. At you local five and dime get the best, heaviest duty loose-leaf notebook you can buy, spare no expense, because it will get a lot of usage and will need to stand up a long time. Also buy some blank section separators and blank labels. Presumably you already have plenty of typing paper (8½ x 11). You will need it punched to go into the notebook. If you wish you can purchase a small hand punch and punch each sheet a hole at a time. My suggestion is to take the package of paper to a local printer and they will create your holes for you at a nominal cost. You can buy prepunched paper, of course, but it is not always available. The paper you use should be medium weight. It must be strong enough to withstand a lot of wear, yet thin enough to create as little bulk as possible. The manual will get pretty large and thick before you finish.

Each person does his/her work at home. Write up each item as clearly as you know how. If you need to, clip out pictures from journals or supply catalogs to demonstrate your specific instruments or tools. You can draw diagrams or sketch instruments or cabinet or tray layouts. Then after you've finished each item, bring it into the office and let the others read it and edit it for clarity. After all, it will be of little use if it is not understandable to others.

Once a section is finished and has been edited, it should be typed. If each of you can type your own section, so much the better. Otherwise you'll have a terrific burden placed on the secretary to try to type it all. Using two or three different typewriters and type faces isn't usually of too much concern, but naturally it will look nicer if it is all done on the same machine.

If you are using pictures, clippings, diagrams, examples of charts, slips and the like, you will probably want to glue these onto the pages. If you do, make sure you keep the glue minimized, and I would suggest that you let it dry overnight heavily pressed with several books. The gluing tends to wrinkle the pages and will make the manual thicker than necessary.

At this time do not attempt to number the pages. Be careful to keep them in order, however, if you have a section running over several sheets. A lightly penciled numbering system will help keep such in line at this point.

After you finally have all the sections properly typed up and glued, you are ready to assemble the manual. This should be done with some organization in mind. Place the more-likely-to-be-used items in the beginning of each section, and those less likely to be needed toward the rear.

Now you can number the pages consecutively. It would be best and easier for each "author" to do her own section, page one through whatever. Then you will have no heavy burden on any one person.

Each major division will then start with page one and you'll need individual tables of contents at the beginning of each division. If you wish you can construct a final, complete table of contents in the very beginning of the book also, but this is actually superfluous.

The Follow-Through

After you finally have the manual, do not just breathe a sigh of relief and stick it off in a corner somewhere. It will have been a great benefit to all of you just putting it together in the sense of learning more about each other's jobs and tasks, likes and dislikes, and certainly a project like this creates a great *esprit de corps.* But to really use it to its proper end, you should take it out every month or so at office conferences and read a section or two out of it. In this way you will all stay reasonably familiar with each other's areas.

Remember, too, that ideas change, and you may add new duties or delete old ones. Your manual should be continually updated in order to remain helpful. If your doctor buys a new piece of equipment, you'll need a page on its operation and care. You'll need a note about when and where it was purchased and what to do if it malfunctions, and where in the office the warranty is filed. This page should be numbered according to its relative importance in the manual—not just stuck in the end. You should number it in the consecutive order as 3a, or 7c, or whatever. Then you can add any number of pages between the original page 7 and page 8 without messing up your entire numbering system. If you should run out of "as" and "bs," go to "aa," and "bb," etc. You will need to add these additional pages onto the table of contents at the beginning of the section, so some retyping may be necessary here. If you have triple spaced the original table of contents, you can easily add two pages between each page before needing to retype the entire table.

18 | *Time and Work-Saving Tips*

How to Handle Salesmen

As you know, your office is frequented by all kinds of salesmen day after day. As much as your dentist might want to do so, he simply doesn't have the time to spend listening to and talking with each man. This is where you, the efficient dental secretary, can be tremendous benefit to all concerned.

What you should do it this: allow no salesmen to see the doctor. In this way you will be fair to all of them (or is it unfair to all?). You politely greet each one and when he asks to see the dentist you inform him he is with a patient. You need not say he cannot be disturbed, just let the salesman assume this.

Ask the detail man the name of his company or ask for a card. Then tell him the doctor will not be able to see him today, but if he cares to tell you what he has to offer, and will leave any printed matter, you will relay this to the dentist. Then when the doctor has had an opportunity to look the material over, if he is interested, you will contact the salesman for a convenient appointment to return and discuss it with the doctor.

You therefore become the main person the salesman needs to see and he will give you all necessary information. It is not up to you to decide on or edit the material. You should not pass word to the dentist that you are favorably or unfavorably impressed with the man or the product. Let the doctor receive from you a straightforward report on who, what, etc. Then he can make a clear-cut decision on just whom or what he wants to follow through on and have you contact later for an appointment with the salesman.

Be sure to request all the pertinent literature the detail man has to offer, and if he has any price list, request this also.

Naturally, you must realize that in order to properly follow through with this procedure, it behooves you to know as much about what the detail man describes as possible, so please keep on your toes. Read the current journals and know what specific equipment and drugs are for and how they are to be used even if you are the dental secretary and only rarely enter the treatment rooms.

Periodically you should ask your employer if there is anything that he particularly wishes to learn about. You then have the opportunity to look through your file of business cards for the name and address of a detail man who might have that information. You then contact him and gather the information as usual and present this to the dentist. If he still wants more help, you can arrange a specific conference for the doctor with the salesman.

Incidentally, since salesmen frequently seem to move from job to job, you'd better keep your "salesman file" set up on a company-by-company alphabetical basis, rather than by the salesman's name. This way you can contact the company easily instead of trying to find a salesman who is no longer with that particular company.

Many of the dental journals, formal as well as informal, have enclosed within them printed cards for additional information from advertisers. It would be helpful for your doctor if you read these ads also (in addition to the educational literature) and look for items you may have heard your dentist mention. If you see something you or one of the other auxiliaries may be interested in also, you can fill out the information request card and send it in. All of this will help your doctor as well as the staff stay up-to-date.

Babysitting Problems in the Dental Office

Nothing can disturb an afternoon quite so much as a reception room with a couple of boisterous tots waiting for mother to get her teeth cleaned. For some reason parents seem to think the kids will behave better when she's only having a prophy than when she's having operative dentistry performed. She wouldn't think of bringing them if she were anticipating, say, an extraction, but a "minor" appointment seems okay to her. It is all pretty ridiculous, isn't it? Well, anyway here they are and you're busy and what do you do?

If your office has an audiovisual machine of any sort, try to get the kids to watch the "movie." Most AV companies have film-strips geared to younger children, and these work pretty well. They will run eight to ten minutes and occupy them for a while. If you have two or three, so much the better—you can get most of your own work done anyway. Even if your films are geared to adults, you can frequently show them to just about any age. I wouldn't let a tot watch a film that showed anything like surgery or needles or forceps or such, but even if they do not understand it all, they'll frequently watch. It's almost like the lousy TV commercial, you've seen it a hundred times, it's boring, it's irrelevant, but you watch it because it is something to do. And who knows, maybe a four-year-old wants to know about root canal therapy!

No audiovisual? Okay, next we try comic books and wee tot picture books. You do not really want to have a reception room cluttered with frayed comic books (unless your doctor is a pedodontist). So, keep a stack handy, but not in the reception room. Issue no more than two books to a child so as to keep them under some control. Explain that after they've looked at these, they can turn them in to you and you'll swap them for some more.

Having coloring books and crayons available is quite helpful, but be sure to have a reasonable place for the little darlings to work, and keep a close eye on them. Otherwise you may need to wash up some walls or flooring or lamp shades. Regular coloring books are inexpensive at local stores. Also, you may want to purchase special dental coloring books that are available. These are more costly than others, and are rather meaningless to the younger children, so make your selections accordingly. Incidentally, boys generally don't like to color pictures of dolls or clothes; girls don't prefer tanks, ships and rockets either.

If you can do so, go to a local toy store and purchase several simple toys—for boys and girls. These could be puzzles, or a small wooden train, or a small doll house with furniture. These are inexpensive and yet they will consume a great deal of their time.

Naturally, the best solution is to head off the problem in the beginning. If you have any inkling that mom is going to bring the kids, you must try to convince her that it is not in *their* best interest to do so. Politely and as subtly as possible, let her know you will not be able to babysit and that it is a *severe* imposition in the office to have them here. Naturally you will not want to offend her, but simply pass the word.

Frequently Mom will schedule (or try to) herself and one or two kids all in one morning with the hygienist, or even the doctor. Don't let her. What happens is that each child is acceptable while he is in the chair, but once out, he's ready to go, and cannot because his sister or mother is in the chair. He gets restless, tired, boisterous. Then sister comes out and the two of them wait for Mother and the entire situation gets worse in a geometric progression.

Your task is to thoroughly convince Mother that it is emotionally bad for the little dears to treat them this way. It is very important that all possible thoughts about dentistry be pleasant, and waiting is never pleasant. When thinking of what is best for the child, he should be scheduled so as to come, be treated and leave promptly. True, it is somewhat of an inconvenience for Mother, but after all we certainly want to do what is best for the child so he will not grow up with fears and unfounded dread about dentistry, In this way you place the burden on Mother to help the child and she is much more likely to follow through than if you state simply and dogmatically that the doctor will not permit unattended children in the office.

Those Dental Meetings

If your dentist goes to a lot of dental meetings, you may find yourself with a lot of "free" time on your hands. These periods can be totally wasted or can be utilized to a real advantage.

If you care about your office and your doctor, you will use this time to clean or freshen up the office. You are probably too busy to give the office a thorough cleaning during the regular busy schedule, so now you have time. Start at the top shelf and remove every item, dust it, dust the shelf and replace it. Remember, even closed cabinets pick up dust.

After completely finishing this chore (and it is certainly a chore, but an imporant one) you should go through all of the dental cabinets and resterilize the instruments and replace them. A layer of dust can easily spread over all the tools and this is not a good thing.

You can follow through by cleaning and vacuuming the chairs and units. In other words use the time to do things that (1) you would not have time to do otherwise, and (2) would thoroughly disrupt the office.

If your doctor has no objections, make arrangements with a janitorial service to come in and clean. Have them clean out all ceiling light fixtures, wash the walls, shampoo the carpets, clean and wax the floors, and wash the windows.

Along this line, if your doctor plans any redecoration soon, this would be a great time for the painters.

If you haven't had time to do so recently, go through the patient's charts and unmount and discard old, out-of-date X-rays. You may wish to discard old financial records, or go through the files and remove inactive and "dead" charts to another spot.

If there are several auxiliaries on the staff, your doctor may prefer (he probably will not insist) that one or two of you take some of your vacation then. He will probably want to have the telephone covered (answered regularly), so schedule to keep one assistant present. This may be no problem if a telephone answering service is available though.

If you and the other auxiliaries attend the dental meetings, you have certain obligations to your doctor. The top of these is to learn as much as you can while there. If you are the true professional you should be, you will want to do this without any suggestions. Go around to all of the booths and talk to the salesmen there. Look at every single item they have on display.

Certainly there may be thousands, but you just might see something new that your doctor may want to know about.

Pick up any give-away literature available and bring it back home to the doctor. Certainly sign up for or pick up any free samples offered.

If possible take notes during the lectures you attend. If the doctor is there with you, you can help refresh his memory when he returns home. If he is not there, you can tell him what you learned and maybe help him in this way. The better DAs keep complete files with typed notes about every meeting.

Dental meetings have a bad habit of becoming strictly social, and along with this goes gossip. Please do not do your doctor the disservice of talking about him or his practice in a detrimental or gossipy manner. You are free to listen to others talk about their boss' personal life or problems, but your colleagues (and your doctor) will have nothing but total respect and envy for your honesty and real professionalism when they discover you will not talk about your boss.

Following through with this view, please don't repeat what you hear, even to your boss or husband. If you do help spread gossip it will place you on as low a level as those who started it.

The Staff Conference

Throughout this book much has been mentioned about the staff meetings or conference. This is a vital part or key to success to the well-oiled machine. It is here that you all can discuss various problems and ways to approach them in an unhurried, uninterrupted manner.

The conference time should be scheduled so there are likely to be no interruptions. Frequently a good time is to set it over an extended lunch period. Schedule as long as necessary with no patients coming, take the telephone off the hook, lock the door and place a note on it stating when the office will reopen, and go to it.

If you have a conference at regular intervals, and this is best, each party can gather a list of items they want to discuss and present them at the appropriate time.

The conference should be rather formalized at least to the

extent of having an agenda. After the first one, start first with old business to clear up, then start on new problems.

The secretary should keep accurate notes and minutes and these should be read at the subsequent meetings. This gets everyone back into the train of thought they were in at the last meeting.

Generally the dentist will use the first part of the conference for declaring any changes he wishes to make in procedure. As she is usually aware of these as she works constantly with him, the chairside assistant probably already knows these changes, but it is important for all of the staff to be aware of them. If any of these changes need to be added to the office manual, it can be done accordingly.

Next, one by one, each staff member can bring up a point to ponder and the entire collective body can discuss it and arrive at the best decision.

Care must be used by all parties not to bring personal problems into the conference. If you have a special problem that is bothering you and it doesn't concern the working of the entire office procedure, don't mention it here. Just wait until later and discuss it privately with your employer.

Likewise, personalities must not be allowed to enter the picture. Otherwise the conference can disintegrate into cheap, pointless chatter and become a real waste of time.

Do not use the fact that you may have two or three auxiliaries to the one doctor make you feel you can overpower the doctor with persuasion for some particular item. In this conference the majority may not necessarily rule, because, as has been said before, it is the doctor's office and if he doesn't feel comfortable with a certain procedure he should and will not be forced into it.

On a positive basis all of you should use the conference as an opportunity to further the efficiency of the office, which in turn will better your working conditions. You can help improve employee-employee, and employee-employer relations, and dentist-patient relations.

In summary, if you will consider the real purpose of the office staff conference, and utilize it to its fullest, you will prove time and again that you are truly the professional dental auxiliary.

Index